# Antioxidants
# Vitamins C & E for Health

**The breakthrough.** One of the most important medical advances of the last few decades is a new understanding of the ways by which human body is damaged and weakened, making it susceptible to a wide range of diseases. This entirely new body of knowledge only began to come to light in the early 1970s.

**The knowledge.** The essence of this knowledge is that most diseases result from damage to our body cells and tissues. This damage is caused by enormously destructive chemical groups called free radicals. These free radicals are constantly attacking body proteins cells, and even DNA, causing potentially serious damage. Free radicals have been implicated in some of the most serious conditions, such as heart diseases, strokes, kidney damage, and possibly cancer. They are even partly responsible for human ageing.

**The good news**. Medical research has established that free radicals can be effectively combated. This is where the antioxidant vitamins come in. Free radicals can be limited, and even prevented, by taking large, but perfectly safe, doses of antioxidant vitamins C and E. Anti-oxidants are recognized as one of the most powerful weapons to counter the damage of free radicals. They are of vital importance to our health. They not only offer protection against disease, but also promote good health.

## The Author

Dr Robert Youngson OstJ, MB, Ch.B., DTM&H, DO, F.R.C. Ophth., a former medical consultant, is now a full-time writer. He is the author of more than thirty popular medical and science books including *Living with Asthma, Coping with Hay Fever* and *Coping with Eczema* and has written extensively on medical topics for *Reader's Digest*. He is the author of the *Royal Society of Medicine Encyclopedia of Family Health* and broadcasts frequently on television and radio on health issues.


**How to Order**

This book is also available on special quantity discounts from the publisher Orient Paperbacks, 5A/8 First Floor, Ansari Road, Darya Ganj, New Delhi - 110 002. Tel: +91-11-2327 8877, Fax: +91-11-2327 8879 email: mail@orientpaperbacks.com. On your business letterhead, kindly include information concerning the intended use of the books and the number of copies you wish to purchase.

# Antioxidants
## Vitamins C and E for Health

Dr. Robert Youngson

Orient Paperbacks
DELHI | MUMBAI | HYDERABAD

*To Heather*



www.orientpaperbacks.com

ISBN 13: 978-81-222-0269-4

1st Published 2000
5th Printing 2011

*Antioxidants: Vitamins C and E for Health*



Published in arrangement with
Sheldon Press, England

Cover design by Vision Studio

The logo and trademark 'Good Health First' are owned by Orient Paperbacks, a division of Vision Books Pvt. Ltd.

Published by
**Orient Paperbacks**
(A Division of Vision Books Pvt. Ltd.)
5A/8 Ansari Road, New Delhi-110 002

Printed in India at
Ravindra Printing Press, Delhi-110 006

# Contents

# Introduction

One of the most important medical advances of the last decades of the twentieth century is a new understanding of the way in which a wide range of diseases and other agencies cause damage to the human body. This is entirely new knowledge that only began to come to light in the early 1970s. As in the case of many important advances, interest in it began slowly and, at first, only a scattering of professional scientific reports on the subject appeared. But as more and more evidence accumulated from research, the literature has grown steadily, and in the last five years or so it has suddenly erupted. Today, many hundreds of papers are appearing on the matter in all the major medical journals.

The essence of all this research is that the damage to our cells and tissues that is at the root of most diseases is caused by highly active and dangerous chemical groups called 'free radicals'. Free radicals are constantly being formed in the body as a result of basic disease processes. They are also formed following exposure to cigarette smoke, car exhaust, industrial fumes and almost all forms of radiation. The destructive effect of free radicals on tissues and organs is very serious. They play an important part role in the production of atherosclerosis – the cause of coronary heart disease, strokes and gangrene – the number one killer in the Western world. They are implicated in the development of cancer and many other disease groups. They are even partly responsible for human ageing.

All this would be of academic interest only were it not for the fact that a great deal of research has shown that free radicals can be effectively combated. This is where antioxidant vitamins come in. It has now been established that the damaging effects of free radicals can be limited or even prevented by taking large, but perfectly safe, doses of the antioxidant vitamins C and E. High body levels of vitamin E, for instance, have been proved to substantially reduce mortality from coronary heart disease.

Antioxidant vitamins are now recognized as being of considerable importance to health. Unfortunately, outside scientific and medical circles the subject of free radicals and antioxidant vitamins is not widely understood. The medical press has, so far, been careful to avoid exaggerated claims, but the importance of the matter is being increasingly recognized. It is now time that the real facts were presented in a form that everyone can understand. That is the purpose of this book. This is not, like many popular medical books, yet another unsustainable miracle claim or just another piece of pseudo-science written by a journalist. Free radicals and antioxidants are important to all of us and this book shows you why. It also offers you the opportunity to do something for yourself to promote your own health.

# 1
# Why Antioxidants?

If, say 30 years ago, you had asked a top medical scientist to tell you what the items in the following list had in common, he or she would have been hard pressed to give you an answer:

- Heart attack;
- Angina;
- Heart failure;
- Stroke;
- Ageing;
- Brain damage;
- Kidney disease;
- Cancer;
- Cataract;
- Poisoning;
- Radiation sickness;
- Rheumatoid arthritis;
- Male infertility;
- Retinopathy of prematurity;
- Malnutrition;
- Common cold.

Today we have the answer. All these conditions are either caused or contributed to by free radicals. Free radicals can do you a lot of harm. If your body fails to combat them effectively, they will kill you. We now know that in most of the major diseases that kill people prematurely or ruin the quality of their lives, the actual bodily damage is caused by free radicals.

These short-lived but enormously damaging chemical groups are constantly attacking body proteins, carbohydrates, fats and DNA, causing potentially serious damage unless checked. In this sense, the body really is a battlefield. Scientists believe that, on average, every cell in your body suffers around 10,000 free radical hits each day. And each of these hits can set up a chain reaction that can kill a cell. Needless to say, the body strikes back, as we shall see. There is no way you can avoid free radicals, but there is a lot you can do to cut down the numbers produced in your body and to ensure that the maximum number of those that are produced are neutralized before they can do you harm.

## *Linus Pauling and antioxidants*

The antioxidant vitamin story really starts with the great American chemist, Linus Pauling (1901–94), who won the Nobel Prize twice and was one of the most distinguished scientists of the twentieth century. His book, *The Nature of the Chemical Bond and the Structure of Molecules and Crystals*, revolutionized chemistry and was described as one of the most influential science texts ever written. He played a foremost part in laying the foundations of modern chemistry, biochemistry and molecular biology. He adapted chemistry to quantum mechanics and pioneered several fundamentally new ways of working out the structure of molecules. *New Scientist* described him as one of the 20 greatest scientists of all time, on a par with Newton, Darwin and Einstein.

In 1970, Pauling published a book called *Vitamin C and the Common Cold* in which he expressed the opinion, based on careful observation of his own experience, that regular daily dosage of vitamin C, in amounts well in excess of the minimum required to prevent deficiency, would produce 'an increased feeling of wellbeing, and especially a striking decrease in the number of colds caught, and in their severity'. Pauling was well aware that most of the previous trials of the method had produced disappointing results, but pointed out that in none of the trials had the dosage taken by the participants been nearly large enough. They were, in fact, little more than was needed to prevent vitamin C deficiency.

Pauling's case was that vitamin C had properties over and above those of preventing scurvy, but that if these properties were to be apparent, the amounts taken had to be very large by normal nutritional standards. Pauling made the case that large doses of vitamin C were by no means abnormal. He showed conclusively that, at a time when humans were evolving and were at the hunter-gatherer stage, the amounts of vitamin C taken must often have been very large.

Assuming that early people must have eaten anything edible they could get their hands on, he decided to work out how much vitamin C they would have taken in if, as must often have happened, the total daily calorie requirement (about 2,500 calories) was met from a single foodstuff. The results were surprising. If they had eaten enough peas and beans to get 2,500 calories, they would have taken in 1,000 mg (1 gram) of vitamin C. Vegetables with a low vitamin C content would have provided 1,200 mg; vegetables and fruits with an intermediate content would have provided 3,400 mg; high C foods like cabbage, cauliflower, chives and mustard greens would have provided 6,000 mg per day; and very high C foods like blackcurrants, kale, parsley, peppers and broccoli would have provided no less than 12,000 mg per day.

There are 1,000 mg in a gram, so many people must often have had a daily dose of at least several grams and sometimes about 10 grams. These figures are way above the amount that the nutritionists tell us are required to prevent scurvy. Official figures for daily requirements range between 20 and 60 mg, the higher amounts being required by nursing mothers. Since humans evolved in an environment providing quantities of vitamin C of this order, Pauling inferred that the ideal daily intake for most adults should be somewhere in the range of 2,300 to 9,000 mg. The very large vitamin C intake throughout a large part of the evolutionary period implied that big doses of this vitamin should be regarded as 'natural'.

In spite of his persuasive arguments, Pauling was dismissed by many of his colleagues as a crank. It seems obvious that very few of those who scorned his claims had ever read his book. There was a good reason for this dismissive attitude. Almost from the time that vitamins were first discovered, many people – people who did not understand how vitamins worked – assumed that if a little of something could do you good, a lot must be better. So vitamins came to be regarded as tonics and a large market in vitamin supplements quickly grew up.

This was rightly condemned by scientists and doctors, who

were all well aware that to take more than the very small amount needed to prevent vitamin deficiency diseases was silly, a waste of money and sometimes harmful. This was, and remains, the correct scientific view. So it is not particularly surprising that Linus Pauling, for all his eminence as a scientist, was laughed at. Those who had read *Vitamin C and the Common Cold* were aware that Pauling had made some very cogent points, but his insistence that vitamin C in large doses could prevent colds or reduce their severity was not supported by very strong evidence.

## *What happened next*

Many people who recognized Pauling's status and did not think that he would make foolish claims were, however, impressed. This includes the author of this book who, for the last 20 years or so has virtually reversed his previous tendency to regular severe colds by taking at least a gram of vitamin C every day. The extraordinary results of this regimen, of course, led me to take a special interest in vitamin C. So it was with considerable interest that I began to realize, some ten years ago, that something new and very important was quietly emerging in the medical literature.

This was nothing less than a body of growing evidence that the frequency of a wide range of disorders – not just the common cold – could be substantially reduced by taking vitamin C. What had really happened was that, for the first time, we were beginning to understand the real cause of much of the bodily damage featured in various diseases – what doctors call the 'pathology'. This was, we now learned, being caused by a process called 'oxidation'. I will explain oxidation and its causes shortly. The point to be made, at this stage, is that vitamin C has long been known to be a powerful antioxidant – a substance that prevents or controls oxidation.

The literature in the medical journals on biological oxidation and the use of antioxidants has been growing steadily for a decade. This growth has accelerated and in the last four or five years the topic has become commonplace. Many hundreds of papers have now been published in journals like the *Lancet*, the *British Medical Journal*, the *New England Journal of Medicine* and the *Journal of the American Medical Association*. The interest has been so great that there has even been at least one completely new journal devoted exclusively to the subject. The general scientific journals like *Nature* and *Science*, specialized biochemical and molecular biology journals, and the popular science magazines like *New Scientist* and *Scientific American* have also published much material on this subject.

A glance at the further reading section at the end of this book will give some indication of the size of the interest in the subject. This list is only a tiny selection of the enormous number of papers now being published on antioxidants and on the chemical groups – the free radicals – that cause the oxidation damage. In addition, it is now common to come across references to free radical action in papers not primarily concerned with this matter.

Vitamin C is not the only antioxidant vitamin. The others are vitamin E and vitamin A. Note, however, that for practical, safe, antioxidant purposes, only vitamins C and E should be considered suitable. All the members of the B group of vitamins are co-enzymes – necessary for the proper activation of various biochemical reactions, and have nothing to do with oxidation control. Taking more than the minimum requirement serves no useful purpose. Vitamins A and D also have no safe usable antioxidant properties and to take more than the recommended daily allowance is not only wasteful, but can be harmful. This is important.

Very large doses of vitamin A cause chronic poisoning featuring:

- skin dryness, itching and peeling;
- drowsiness, irritability and an irresistible desire to sleep;
- headache;
- loss of appetite;
- enlargement of the liver and spleen;
- painful and tender swellings over the bones.

The vitamin accumulates in the body and the effects take weeks to wear off. Eskimos and their husky dogs never eat polar bear liver (which contains huge quantities of vitamin A) because they know of these effects. One gram of polar bear liver contains up to

12 mg of retinol – 12 times the minimum daily requirement. Vitamin A is also dangerous to the fetus if taken by the mother in doses of 7 to 12 mg a day during the first three months of pregnancy. This can cause congenital abnormalities.

Too much vitamin D causes calcium to be deposited in the kidneys, arteries and other tissues – a serious matter that can lead to all sorts of problems, including kidney failure. Once again, here is a warning about the fallacy of believing that if something is good for you, a lot of it will be even better. This is often true, but you should not count on it. In some cases, a lot is very much worse for you.

You may well have been led astray by journalistic hype and by the use in popular medical literature of the buzzword 'ACE' for vitamins A, C and E. Vitamin A, or more precisely its provitamin beta-carotene, does have antioxidant powers but this vitamin should not, for obvious reasons, be regarded as being in the same category, for antioxidant purposes, as vitamins C and E. It is, of course, important for you to have the minimum amounts of vitamins A and D so as to avoid deficiency diseases. But these amounts can almost always be obtained from a normal, healthy balanced diet.

The basis of the new knowledge is that, in disease and injury, body tissue damage by oxidation is caused by chemical groups known as free radicals. These are used by certain scavenging cells of the immune system – the phagocytes – to destroy unwanted waste material. But they are also produced in enormous numbers in the body when people suffer virus and bacterial infections, smoke cigarettes, or expose themselves to ultraviolet light from the sun and to other forms of radiation.

Produced in excess and not checked, the destructive effect of free radicals on the molecules from which body cells are made, and thus on many tissues and organs, can be very serious. Their importance rests in the fact that they are implicated in such a wide range of diseases. Their role in the two disease groups that are the principal cause of death and disability – heart disease and cancer – is now well understood. This is, by itself, a major medical advance that has already begun to have an important impact on the understanding of disease processes. But the evidence that antioxidant substances such as vitamin C and vitamin E can limit the damaging effects of excess free radicals is even more important.

To quote A.T. Diplock, Professor of Biochemistry at Guy's and St Thomas' Hospitals, London:

> Compelling evidence is now emerging from prospective studies begun in the early 1970s that low dietary intake of vitamin E is indeed a significant risk factor in the aetiogenesis of both ischaemic heart disease and cancer at certain sites. Several prospective studies have shown a correlation between a low dietary level of vitamin C and a high incidence of cardiovascular disease and cancer.

'Aetiogenesis' just means 'cause and origin'. Translated into ordinary language, Professor Diplock's statement means that scientific trials have proved that people who do not take enough vitamin E and vitamin C are more likely to get heart attacks and certain kinds of cancers. And now that we know that these vitamins act, in this context, by their antioxidant powers, it becomes clear that this really is a case in which more than a little of a good thing can be even better.

So now we must take a look at exactly what free radicals are and how antioxidants can deal with them

# 2

# How Free Radicals and Oxidation Harm Your Health

Unless you know a bit about science, you will probably find this chapter difficult in places. A subject like this cannot be adequately covered without a few technicalities, and here I am dealing with the basic scientific facts underlying the whole matter. You might be tempted to skip some of it, but I recommend that you have a go at the whole explanation. It may not turn out to be so bad as you expect. If you do work through it, you will be able to read the rest of this book with a clearer understanding, and you will also be able to take a more critical and intelligent interest in magazine and newspaper articles on the subject.

## *Free radicals*

Medical interest in free radicals is very recent, but chemists have known all about them and have been studying them closely for about 50 years. When they were first proposed about 100 years ago, most chemists were outraged and protested that they were impossible. Gradually, however, they came to realize that free radicals were very real and were fleetingly involved in many important chemical reactions, such as the formation of plastics (polymers), the perishing of rubber and the deterioration of stored foodstuffs. Most free radicals exist only for very short periods before attacking other substances and being neutralized in the process. They can, however, be produced as quickly as they disappear and when they do attack they can turn other substances into free radicals and so set up very damaging chain reactions.

So, what are they? To answer that question we must go back to a few very basic scientific facts.

## *Atoms*

Some free radicals are among the smallest things that exist. One of them consists of a single atom, others of two atoms linked together. Some are larger. Those that we are mainly interested in each consist of two atoms linked together. But, as we shall see, these are not just ordinary atoms. They are atoms with one very special property that makes all the difference to their significance to us. To make this plain, we must take a brief look at atoms in general.

As you know, everything is made of atoms. In chemistry, atoms do not break up but remain intact, even in a chemical reaction as violent as an explosion. Every atom has a central part called the 'nucleus' and a number of tiny particles, called 'electrons', buzzing around it. That's all. The rest is empty space. A vacuum. The nucleus is charged positive and the electrons are charged negative, and there are the same number of electrons as there are positive charges on the nucleus. So the atom, as a whole, has no charge because all the positive charges are neutralized by the negative charges. The electrons occupy regions around the nucleus known as 'orbitals'. Each orbital can hold only two electrons and these are spinning in opposite directions. An orbital with two electrons is stable; an orbital with only one electron is highly unstable.

Atoms differ in the number of electrons they have. There are 92 different kinds of atom in nature, from hydrogen which is the lightest to uranium which is the heaviest, and scientists have made a dozen more. Substances made of collections of atoms of one kind only are called 'elements'. So there are 92 natural elements. Hydrogen has one electron; uranium has 92. So hydrogen has a problem. With only one electron, how does it achieve a stable, two-electron orbital? It solves this problem very quickly, simply by linking up with another hydrogen atom to form a pair that share a filled, two-electron orbital.

## *Molecules*

Most substances are made from a combination of different kinds of atoms linked together. These combinations of atoms are called molecules and they may be quite small or very large – containing a few atoms or many. The molecule of hydrogen consists of two hydrogen atoms linked together. Water consists of an oxygen atom linked to two hydrogen atoms ($H_2O$). Common salt (NaCl) consists of an atom of the metal sodium linked to an atom of the gas chlorine. Other molecules, such as those of proteins or plastics, are very large and may contain hundreds, thousands or even millions of atoms, usually of just a few varieties, all linked together.

Substances made of molecules are called 'compounds' and most of these contain just a few different kinds of atoms. Human beings are made from just over 20 different atoms, but 93.3% of our bodies are made from only four atoms – carbon, hydrogen, oxygen and nitrogen.

## *Atomic bonds*

The way that atoms link together was largely worked out by Linus Pauling, and this provides another association with this great man, because the linkage of atoms is basic to the subject of this book. When atoms join to each other to form molecules they do so by sharing their outer electrons in various ways. These linkages are called 'bonds'. Some atoms can link to only one other atom; some can link to two; some to three; some to four. A single atom of the element carbon can link to four other atoms such as hydrogen, or can link to other carbon atoms. This gives almost infinite possibilities of combinations and permutations, and is the reason why the chemistry of carbon is a complete science in its own right – a science known as 'organic chemistry'. Carbon atoms can link together in long chains, with other kinds of atoms hooked on, or they can link together in rings of six atoms (benzene rings) or in different-sized rings with other atoms.

If a carbon atom links to fewer than the full number of atoms it is capable of linking to, it forms links called 'double bonds' or 'triple bonds'. Contrary to what you might think, double and triple bonds are weaker than single bonds because the carbon atom likes to have all its four bonds properly used up in a stable situation. Compounds with only single bonds are said to be 'saturated'; those with double bonds are 'unsaturated'. Saturated fats, for instance, are those containing fatty acids with no double carbon atom bonds. These are the most stable kinds of fats. Unsaturated fats have double bonds and are more easily broken up.

## *Large molecules and small clusters*

Most organic molecules – those found in living things or their products – are fairly large. All of them are based on carbon and many contain only carbon and hydrogen atoms, linked up in chains or rings. Most organic molecules consist of a basic structure of carbon atoms to which small clusters of other atoms are attached. These clusters, or chemical groups, are very important in chemistry, especially in biochemistry – the chemistry of living things – as different groups are responsible for most of the different chemical properties of the molecules.

A long time ago, chemists discovered that when chemical reactions occurred these little clusters, instead of breaking up to release the individual atoms of which they are made, tended to act almost like molecules in their own right, retaining their group identity and linking on, in their entirety, to other molecules. They did not, however, persist for any length of time on their own but always tried to tie themselves on to a molecule. So chemists decided to give these groups a name and called them 'radicals'. This word has no deep hidden meaning. It simply comes from the Latin word *radix*, meaning 'a root', and was selected because the atom cluster hangs from the molecule like a root and can 'root' itself in other molecules.

As you have probably guessed, free radicals are radicals that are temporarily unattached to a molecule. Unattached radicals are not happy just to sit around like the more stable molecules of compounds; rather they are constantly looking for something to latch on to. Many of them are quite small, consisting of only two or three atoms; some are larger. The one thing they all have in common is that they are remarkably active. As we shall see, some of the common forms of free radicals are highly dangerous to our bodies.

## *The unpaired electron*

We must now look at the way in which the atoms of water are bonded together. Remember that water consists of a single atom of oxygen with two hydrogen atoms linked on to it. The bonds between the oxygen atom and each hydrogen atom consist of a pair of electrons shared between the atoms – one from the hydrogen atom and one from the oxygen atom. The water molecule, however, routinely separates into two particles called 'ions' that wander about freely. The term 'ion' just means 'wanderer'.

One of these two ions of water is a hydrogen atom (H) without its electron. Bearing in mind that the nucleus of an atom is positively charged and that electrons are negative, you will see that this ion is positively charged. The other ion is a complete hydrogen atom, with its electron, linked to a complete oxygen atom but with the electron missing from the first hydrogen atom also stuck on (OH). So this ion is negatively charged. The H ion is called a 'positive ion', and the OH ion is called a 'negative ion'. This is the normal way for water to be split up and is known as 'ionization'. Positive and negative ions are important in chemistry, and many chemical reactions occur between different ions coming together.

About 50 years ago it was discovered to the astonishment of the chemists that, under certain circumstances, the water molecule can split up in another, quite different, way. If, for instance, water is exposed to radiation such as X-rays or gamma rays, the two-electron bonds between the oxygen and the hydrogen atoms can briefly split, leaving one electron on the hydrogen and one on the oxygen atom combination – the hydroxyl radical – thus creating two radicals, both electrically neutral but both having only one spare electron. Thus, momentarily, we have two atoms each with only one electron in an outer orbital. Both the hydrogen radical and the hydroxyl radical are horribly active. It is the unpaired electron that makes them so chemically active. A group with an unpaired electron is highly unstable and is desperate either to pick up another electron from somewhere, or to give up its solitary electron. The hydroxyl radical is the most reactive free radical known to chemistry and will attack almost every molecule in the body.

Nature likes things to be stable. Hydrogen atoms, which have only one electron, never exist individually for more than a fraction of a second but immediately join up in pairs to produce a hydrogen molecule of two atoms with a stable pair of electrons ($H_2$). The same applies to a hydrogen radical – which is, of course, simply an isolated hydrogen atom. It is this stable, two-electron, state that free radicals are always aiming for, and if a free radical is formed, it will at once attack the nearest molecule – whatever it may be – to steal or hand over an electron and achieve stability. This can have very serious effects.

So now you know exactly what a free radical is. It is any atom or group of atoms that can exist independently and that contains at least one unpaired electron. Some free radicals are stabilized by their peculiar structure and exist for appreciable lengths of time. But the great majority have only a very brief independent existence before either grabbing an extra electron or giving one up. Not all free radicals are small, like the hydrogen or hydroxyl radicals. The methyl radical has a carbon atom and three hydrogen atoms; the ethyl radical has two carbons and five hydrogens. Some are large and complex, containing rings of carbon atoms (benzene rings) and various side chains. All, however, have a single, unpaired, electron somewhere.

## *Free radical chain reactions*

From the medical point of view we are interested mainly in two free radicals – the hydroxyl radical (-OH) and the superoxide radical which consists of two linked oxygen atoms ($O_2$) with a single, unpaired electron.

These oxygen free radicals, each with their single electron, can attack and damage almost every molecule found in the body. They are so active that, after they are formed, only a small fraction of a second elapses before they join on to something. In so doing they can either hand over their unpaired electron or capture an electron from some other molecule to make up the pair. In either event, the radical becomes stable but the attacked molecule now has an unpaired electron and has thus been converted into a radical. You can see that this is a perfect recipe for starting a chain reaction that will zip destructively and at high speed through a tissue.

Fortunately, the hydroxyl free radical does not normally occur in living systems because of the strength of the bonds linking the hydrogen and oxygen atoms in the water molecules. But if anyone is exposed to ionizing radiation, these bonds can be broken by the radiation so that hydroxyl radicals result. This is what happened to the workers at Chernobyl. It is the basis of radiation sickness – the dreadful, often fatal, damage that occurs in people exposed to large doses of radiation.

If hydroxyl radicals attack DNA, chain reactions run along the DNA molecule causing damage to, and mutations in, the genetic material. These chain reactions can even cause actual breakage of the DNA strands. The body does its best to repair this damage by the natural processes of DNA repair replication, but imperfect repair leaves altered DNA and can give rise to cancer. When strong X-rays or gamma radiation are deliberately used to kill cancers, they do so primarily by producing large numbers of hydroxyl free radicals.

It would be wrong to leave you with the impression that radiation is the only way free radicals are produced, or that free radicals are only produced from water. Radiation is the only common way that hydroxyl free radicals are formed in the body from water. Unfortunately, there are other ways in which hydroxyl radicals can be formed and there are several other kinds of free radicals, especially the superoxide radical, that can be produced in other ways. They are produced by many disease processes, by poisons, drugs, metals, cigarette smoke, car exhaust gases, heat, lack of oxygen, even sunlight. There is much more about this elsewhere in the book.

As we now know, the damage that is done by free radicals features the chemical reaction known as 'oxidation'. Free radical attack on tissue is commonly referred to in the literature as 'oxidative stress'. This idea of oxidation is particularly important and deserves a closer look.

## *Oxidation*

The statement that free radicals act by oxidation might not mean very much to you, but don't worry. The matter is really very simple. Oxidation is a kind of burning and is always damaging to whatever is oxidized. It can be fast or it can be slow.

If a bright iron nail is left outside it will soon rust. If you strike a match and let it burn, the firm white wood turns to a brittle, blackened ash. If you start your car, a little petrol gets turned to a mixture of gases and soot that come out of the exhaust pipe. These are all examples of oxidation. In all these cases the element oxygen – which makes up about 20% of the atmospheric air – links up chemically with the original substance, whether iron, cellulose or hydrocarbon, to form an entirely new compound. If the nail rusts completely – which it will eventually do if exposed to air and water – it turns to a pile of red powdery stuff called 'iron oxide'. When the match and the petrol are oxidized, equally major changes occur in which the carbon, hydrogen and oxygen of which they are made combines with oxygen from the air to form new compounds. These are mostly gases – water vapour (hydrogen and oxygen) and carbon dioxide (carbon and oxygen). The ash of the match and the soot from the exhaust are mostly carbon that has not linked with oxygen to form carbon dioxide.

Although the term 'oxidation' originally meant adding oxygen as in these examples, it has now been extended to have a wider meaning. Chemists now define oxidation as any chemical reaction that involves the loss of an electron from an atom. And, as you have seen, removing electrons from atoms is exactly what free radicals are particularly good at doing.

The whole point about striking matches and burning petrol is to release energy. Oxidation is always associated with a release of energy, usually in the form of heat. Even the rusting of the nail releases heat, but very slowly so we do not usually notice it. The heat from the match is obvious, and that from the petrol expands the gas in the cylinders of the car engine, drives down the pistons and moves the car along. When you eat a McDonald's cheeseburger, it too is oxidized – rather slowly so that the heat energy is released at a suitable rate to keep up your body temperature and supply energy to the cells.

So, although oxidation is obviously important and necessary, it can also be damaging. Releasing energy is always a double-edged weapon. Matches can light the gas, but they can also set fire to a house. Petrol and other active or explosive substances can be used in different ways when they are oxidized, some constructive, some destructive. It is exactly the same with free radicals. The body cannot do without them because they are involved in many essential chemical reactions. But if more free radicals are produced than the body needs, or if the body's methods of coping with free radicals prove inadequate, then we are in trouble.

In that event – and it is happening all the time – we naturally want to try to do something to stop it. This is where 'antioxidants' come in. An antioxidant is any substance that retards or prevents deterioration, damage or destruction by oxidation. In a medical context, antioxidants are comparatively new, but in other branches of science they have been around for a long time.

## *Antioxidants*

For many years, chemists have known that free radical oxidation action can be controlled or even prevented by a range of antioxidant substances. It is, for instance, vital that lubricating oils should remain stable and liquid and should not dry up like paints. For this reason, such oils usually have small quantities of antioxidants, such as phenol or amine derivatives, added to them. Although plastics are often formed by free radical action, they can also be broken down by the same process. So they, too, require protection by antioxidants like phenols or naphthols. Low-density polythene is also often protected by carbon black to absorb ultraviolet light which would otherwise cause free radical production.

Food in storage deteriorates by oxidation. When, for instance, fat goes rancid it does so by a free radical oxidation reaction. Oxidized fats are new compounds that taste and smell horrible and anything that can prevent this happening is of economic importance. So the chemists have for some time been actively looking for antioxidants for this purpose. To date, the most popular antioxidant food additives have been BHA (butylated hydroxyanisole), BHT (butylated hydroxytoluene), propyl gallate and tocopherol (vitamin E). These antioxidants act by donating hydrogen atoms to the hydroxyl radical (see above) so that water is formed. The equation is simple: $H + OH = H_2O$. In other words, two dangerously active radicals combine to form a harmless molecule: water.

Ironically, too, the irradiation of food – which is an excellent way of killing bacteria that can cause spoilage and may be dangerous – can, in itself, cause free radical production that can lead to unacceptable chemical changes in the food. So it may sometimes be necessary to counteract the undesirable effects of irradiation of food by using antioxidants.

## *Natural body antioxidants*

Fortunately, the body has its own antioxidants for damage limitation. One of the most effective of these is the substance tocopherol (vitamin E). This vitamin dissolves in fat and that is especially important because much the most significant free radical damage in the body is damage to the membranes of cells and to low-density lipoproteins (see p. 32) and these are made of fat molecules. Vitamin C is also a powerful antioxidant, but is soluble in water, not in fat. This means that it gets distributed to all parts of the body. The two vitamins are both highly efficient at mopping up free radicals, and sometimes even cooperate in so doing.

Other natural body antioxidants include compounds such as cysteine, glutathione and D-penicillamine, and blood constituents such as the iron-containing molecule transferrin and the protein ceruloplasmin. These act either by preventing free radicals from being produced or by mopping them up. The body also contains a number of important antioxidant enzymes. An enzyme is a highly active protein that accelerates a chemical reaction. Most of what goes on in the body is promoted by thousands of different enzymes.

The most interesting antioxidant enzyme is superoxide dismutase (commonly called SOD by the scientists). There is no reason to be rude about this marvellous enzyme, for we really need it. The discovery of this antioxidant enzyme was one of the events that really got the doctors interested in free radicals. There was tremendous interest in biochemical circles when it was discovered that the enzyme has no other function than to change the dangerous superoxide free radical to the safer hydrogen peroxide. Hydrogen peroxide ($H_2O_2$), although not a free radical, is not particularly pleasant stuff to have around. The extra oxygen atom is readily available to cause oxidation, making it an active compound useful for producing blonde hair. So the body has two other enzymes, catalase and glutathione peroxidase, that break down hydrogen peroxide to water and oxygen.

Each of these three enzymes is made in cells under the instructions of a length of genetic code in DNA. Every cell in our bodies contains the instructions for making these enzymes (to say nothing of thousands of other enzymes). So unless free radicals are important, why would evolution go to such lengths to protect the body against them?

## *How are oxygen free radicals produced in the body?*

Free radicals can originate in body cells in various ways. External radiation, including ultraviolet light, X-rays and gamma rays from radioactive material, is a potent source. Such radiation acts by breaking linkages between atoms, leaving the radicals with their unpaired electrons to do their chain-reaction damage. Free radicals occur in the course of various disease processes. In a heart attack, for instance, when the supply of oxygen and glucose to the heart muscle is cut off, the real damage to the muscle is caused by the vast numbers of free radicals that are produced.

Chemical poisoning of many kinds promotes free radicals, as does excessive oxygen intake from inhaling pure oxygen. The body's necessity to break down a wide range of drugs to safer substances (detoxication) also involves free radical production. The poisonousness (toxicity) of many chemicals and drugs is actually due either to their conversion to free radicals or to their effect in forming free radicals. Inflammation – one of the commonest kinds of bodily disorder – is associated with free radical production, but the free radicals are probably the cause of the inflammation rather than the effect. However, the body actually uses free radicals to kill bacteria within the scavenging cells of the immune system – the phagocytes, and when excessive numbers of these are present in an inflamed area, the free radical load almost certainly adds to the tissue damage, making everything worse. This is probably what happens in rheumatoid arthritis, for instance.

Free radicals also arise in the course of normal internal cellular function. This is called 'metabolism' and it is, of course, essential. Metabolic processes require many chemical reactions that involve free radical action. The joining of chains of amino acids (polymerization) to form proteins, or the polymerization of glucose molecules into the polysaccharide, glycogen, for instance, involve free radical action. In most cases the process is automatically controlled and the number of free radicals does not become dangerously high. Fortunately, the body has, throughout the course of millions of years of evolution, become accustomed to coping with free radicals and has evolved various schemes for doing so. In the course of metabolism, important and potentially dangerous free radicals such as superoxide and hydroxyl radicals are produced.

You can now relax. All the difficult science is over and it is now fairly plain sailing.

# 3
# How Antioxidants Can Protect Your Heart and Brain

Most people are unaware that by far the enormous majority of heart disorders – angina pectoris and heart attacks – are not primarily heart problems. The same goes for the enormous majority of strokes – minor and major – which are not really brain problems. The explanation of this seemingly paradoxical statement is that, in both cases, the trouble is in the arteries that supply the heart and the brain with blood. The heart is a powerful muscle and the brain is a mass of nerve tissue and supporting tissue. Both work very hard and both require a massive and continuous supply of well-oxygenated blood. Without this blood supply which also carries the principal cell fuel, glucose – both the heart and the brain would quickly die.

Blood is supplied via the arteries, so it is of vital concern that these arteries should be healthy and, in particular, unobstructed. Few of us really appreciate how fundamentally important our arteries are. We worry and complain about our joints, backs, lungs, legs, veins, skin, even our waterworks, but seldom, if ever, about our arteries. The truth is that artery trouble is far more serious than any of these other things we complain about.

There are, of course, reasons for this neglect. One is lack of the kind of knowledge that this book will give you. Another is that the partial or total blockage caused by arterial disease has its effect, not on the arteries, but on the organs or parts the arteries supply with blood. So when someone gets terrible calf pain on walking and then notices that a toe has turned black, he or she is apt to think that there is something wrong with the muscles or the toes. Even if a whole leg becomes gangrenous – a very common result of serious disease in the arteries supplying the leg – the unfortunate victim may be unaware of what has caused the disaster.

## *The menace of atherosclerosis*

There are several diseases of arteries, but there is one beside which all the others pale into insignificance. This disease is very common and it is called 'atherosclerosis'. (Note that this is not the same as the old-fashioned term 'arteriosclerosis' which was inaccurate and has now been almost completely abandoned.) Atherosclerosis affects almost everyone in the Western world. It begins in childhood and, in most cases, progresses very slowly throughout life. The degree to which it progresses matters a great deal, for the very simple reason that advanced atherosclerosis furs up the affected artery and reduces the amount of blood that can get through it.

If the blood flow is seriously restricted in the arteries, the organs or parts they supply will suffer disorder or malfunction. If the organ is the heart and the narrowing is excessive, the result is a heart attack, possibly death; if it is the brain, the result is a stroke; if it is a leg, the result is gangrene.

Atherosclerosis affects certain arteries more often than others and is particularly liable to occur in those supplying the heart, the brain and the legs. But it can affect almost any arteries and can lead to dire consequences to the eyes, the kidneys, the intestines, some of the endocrine glands and other parts of the body. Atherosclerosis kills more people than any other single disease or cause. It also has a devastating effect on the quality of life of millions, crippling them with angina pectoris and agonizing leg pain on walking and, in other cases, causing progressive and distressing dementia.

Although we have known for years that there is a relationship between diet and atherosclerosis, it is only recently that it has become apparent that the actual damage to the artery that leads to the dangerous narrowing is caused by free radicals.

## *What is atherosclerosis?*

The arteries are the tough, elastic, thick-walled tubes that carry blood, under fairly high pressure, from the heart to the various parts of the body. This blood is fresh from the lungs where it has picked up a good supply of oxygen and it also carries the body fuel, glucose, from the liver and the intestines. Both oxygen and glucose are essential for life and health. The brain and the heart are especially sensitive to lack of oxygen and glucose. If the supply of these vital substances is cut off for more than a few minutes death, or severe brain or heart damage, is inevitable. After the oxygen and glucose have been supplied to the tissues, the blood returns to the heart by way of the low-pressure, thin-walled veins to complete the circulation.

Atherosclerosis affects only arteries, not veins. It is a degenerative disease that starts in the first year of life with fatty streaks in the linings of the arteries. These are present in almost all Western world children and are believed to be the first stage in the process. The most important feature of atherosclerosis is the formation of plaques. These are white or yellowish-white raised areas on the inner surface of the arteries, varying in size from about a third of a centimetre (one-eighth of an inch) across to one and a half centimetres (just over half an inch) across. In severe cases the plaques are so numerous that they run together to form large masses. These plaques have an outer zone of mixed fibrous tissue, scavenging phagocyte cells and abnormal numbers of muscle cells, and a core consisting of a disorganized mass of cell debris and fatty tissue, mainly cholesterol. Around the edges of the plaques are many tiny abnormal blood vessels that have budded out from the wall of the artery.

## *How does atherosclerosis cause harm?*

The arteries most commonly and severely affected by atherosclerosis are the main arterial trunk of the body – the aorta – and its immediate branches. In particular, atherosclerosis affects the coronary arteries – the two branches of the aorta that supply the heart muscle itself with blood; the branches that run down to supply the legs; and the carotid branches than run up the neck to supply the brain and their branches that form a network under the brain. Although the branches to the kidneys and intestines are usually spared, it is common for the openings in the aorta for these branches to be severely narrowed by atherosclerosis.

Arteries are not usually closed off completely by plaques. What happens is that the surface of plaques becomes rough and sometimes broken down (ulcerated). This allows the blood to contact the underlying tissue. Blood is designed to clot whenever it comes in contact with body tissue other than blood vessel linings. So clotting on top of atheromatous plaques is very common. This is called 'thrombosis' and, of course, such a clot can readily close off the artery altogether. Coronary artery thrombosis is the principal cause of heart attacks; cerebral artery thrombosis causes strokes with all their frightening consequences of paralysis, speech and vision disturbance and general disablement. Even more serious strokes occur if small brain arteries are so damaged and weakened by atherosclerosis that they burst. The resulting bleeding around or into the brain is called 'cerebral haemorrhage' and the effects are usually devastating.

Apart from the risk to the brain, heart and other organs, the damage to the aorta itself commonly leads to weakening of the wall and the pressure of the blood in this vessel is so high that the result is often a dangerous ballooning out of the aorta – a condition known as aneurysm. It is hardly necessary to state that an aortic aneurysm is a highly dangerous condition and that the consequences of bursting hardly bear thinking about.

You will see from all this that severe atherosclerosis is a condition to be avoided at all costs. Any knowledge about the ways in which it comes about is valuable knowledge, and any measures that could retard the progress of the disease are priceless. That knowledge now exists and there is good reason to believe that we do have ways of limiting the worsening of this dreadful condition. Forget any ideas you may have that this is simply a matter of cutting down your intake of cholesterol. That simplistic idea has been around for far too long, and there is more to it than that, as we shall see. Cholesterol is an essential body ingredient. Every cell contains cholesterol, and each day a large amount of cholesterol comes down your bile duct from your liver, where it is synthesized, and is reabsorbed into your blood.

Certainly, a reduced intake of saturated fats is a good thing, but there is always plenty of cholesterol in your body to be laid down in the atherosclerotic plaques, if the process that leads to this dangerous deposition is operating. Happily, we are now beginning to understand this process and we know that free radicals are deeply involved.

## *How do free radicals cause atherosclerosis?*

Cholesterol and other fatty materials (lipids) are transported around in the bloodstream in the form of tiny fatty bodies known as 'lipoproteins'. These are loose chemical combinations of fats and proteins. They come in two main kinds, the low-density lipoproteins (LDLs) and the high-density lipoproteins (HDLs). The density comes from the proportion of protein present. HDLs have a lot of protein and a little cholesterol; LDLs have a lot of cholesterol and a little protein. LDLs carry cholesterol and other fats from the liver to the tissues – including the arteries – and HDLs carry cholesterol and fats from the tissues to the liver. You can think of LDLs as the 'baddies' and HDLs as the 'goodies'.

Scientists have known about this for years and have also known that if you eat a lot of saturated fats – stable fats with no double bonds between the carbon atoms, that are solid at room temperature – you will have lots of LDLs in your blood. If you eat only polyunsaturated fats – fats with many double bonds, that are usually liquid at room temperature – you will have far fewer LDLs in your blood. What has not been known is how the cholesterol from the LDLs gets into the atherosclerotic plaques.

## *How lipoproteins become dangerous*

Lipoproteins are not, by themselves, much good at penetrating intact tissue. The way they work is to be taken to the site where their materials are required by blood vessels so tiny that the LDLs are able to get into direct contact with their target cells. Recent research indicates, however, that LDLs that have been attacked by free radicals and oxidized are much more ferocious than normal tame LDLs. Oxidized LDLs can, apparently, fight their way through the inner lining layers of the walls of arteries so that they can deposit their loads under the surface layer.

Some scientists have also proposed that free radicals also act in other ways – by injuring lining cells (endothelium) and smooth muscles cells in the vessel wall; by preventing scavenging cells (phagocytes) from doing their job properly; and by promoting the formation of the large phagocyte foam cells in which the cholesterol accumulates in the plaques. Significantly, research has shown that in rabbits with very high blood cholesterol levels, those given the antioxidant probucol – a drug related to BHT (see p. 24) – develop fewer atherosclerotic plaques than those not given the drug. Probucol has also been used in humans.

So the present view on the production of atherosclerotic plaques is that LDLs do not, unless oxidized, help to form the plaques. Dr Hermann Esterbauer, of the University of Graz, Austria, a foremost researcher in the field of free radical damage to arteries, speaking at a conference at the New York Academy of Sciences on the health implications of vitamin E, stated that there was strong evidence that free radical oxidation of LDLs was the essential fact and that unless LDLs were oxidized they were not capable of forming plaques. Delegates at the conference were told that the natural antioxidants in the LDLs were depleted by the free radicals to the point where they could no longer prevent damaging chain reactions caused by free radicals.

At the same conference, Dr K. Fred Gey of Hoffmann-La Roche, Basel, and a professor at the Institute of Biochemistry and Molecular Biology, University of Berne, reported the results of an interesting survey. This study, co-sponsored by the World Health Organization, investigated the reasons for the striking differences in the mortality, in different countries, from heart disease caused by atherosclerosis of the coronary arteries. It had involved 11,000 men aged 40 to 59 years from 12 countries. In some countries, the death rates from heart disease was much higher than in others. Men living in Scotland and Finland, for instance, were four times as likely to die from heart disease as men living in Italy or Switzerland. There must clearly be some explanation for this remarkable difference, and Dr Gey suggested that it might have been found.

In the course of the survey, the levels of antioxidant vitamin E in the blood of the subjects was monitored over a four-month period. The results were remarkably suggestive. In those with low levels of this vitamin, the death rates were significantly higher than in those with higher levels. This was not a marginal difference. Studies of previous risk factors, such as smoking, high blood pressure and high blood cholesterol, could predict an increased risk of heart disease with an accuracy of only 50%. When the blood levels of these vitamins were also taken into account, the accuracy rose to 94%.

It is probably worth mentioning, in this context, the fact – reported in the *Scottish Medical Journal* in 1989 – that middle-aged Scottish men eat very little fruit and green vegetables. Can this be a pure coincidence?

In 1991, the prestigious weekly journal the *Lancet*, carried a leading article – a report produced by the heart research unit in the Department of Cardiology and Medicine of the University of Edinburgh. This report, by Dr R. A. Riemersma and colleagues, described a research study into whether there was any connection between the levels of certain vitamins in the body and the risk of having angina pectoris. The vitamins concerned were vitamins C, E and A and the substance beta-carotene that is converted by the liver into vitamin A. There was more to this trial than immediately meets the eye.

## *About angina*

Angina pectoris is not, as is commonly thought, a disease, but a symptom. It is the often agonizing tight gripping, constricting pain, 'like a steel band around the chest', that is felt by the sufferer after a certain, often predictable, amount of exertion. Angina usually comes on after walking for a particular distance, comes on more quickly on a cold day or when walking against the wind, and especially when walking uphill. It may be brought on by anxiety or emotion. Sometimes the pain passes down the arms, especially the left arm. Sometimes it radiates through to the back or up into the neck. Altogether it is a very unpleasant and worrying experience.

Angina is worrying because the trouble comes from the heart and is caused by asking the heart to work harder than it comfortably can with the limited oxygen and glucose supply available to it. This supply is limited because the arteries that carry the blood to the heart muscle – the coronary arteries – have been narrowed by atherosclerosis. Atherosclerosis is the disease; angina is the symptom. In the case of most affected people – usually men – the heart can beat away satisfactorily when the person is at rest. But during exertion, the heart has to work harder to pump additional blood to the muscles and there comes a point at which the narrowed coronary arteries cannot supply the needed increase in blood flow. When this happens, the heart complains. Waste materials accumulate around the heart muscle cells and these stimulate pain in the nerve endings. Many people with angina go on like this for years, but in some the condition gradually worsens until it may occur even at rest. In others, the angina becomes more rapidly unstable and there is a serious risk that a coronary artery, or a large branch of it, may become completely blocked, causing coronary thrombosis – a heart attack.

## *Angina and vitamins*

Dr Riemersma's paper was especially interesting for several reasons. First, there is an obvious relationship between angina pectoris and the risk of heart disease; both are caused by the same arterial disorder – atherosclerosis (see p. 29). Second, the vitamins it studied are antioxidants that attack free radicals. Perhaps most interestingly of all, the study – carried out by scientifically very well-informed people – implied a presumption that there might well be a connection between free radicals and heart disease. The results of the study confirmed this presumption. No connection was found between levels of vitamin A and angina. The results for vitamin C were confused by the fact that vitamin C levels are lower in smokers than in non-smokers; and since smoking is an established risk factor for heart disease this could not be attributed to low levels of the vitamin. But so far as vitamin E was concerned, there was no doubt about the result. Even after taking into account smoking, blood pressure, obesity and blood cholesterol levels, the facts were clear. Men with low blood levels of vitamin E were significantly more likely to have angina than men with higher levels.

The authors of the paper concluded that 'some populations with a high incidence of coronary heart disease should supplement their eating habits with more cereals, vitamin E-rich oils, vegetables, and fruit'.

The paper brought out some other very interesting points. As explained above, low-density lipoproteins (LDLs) altered by oxidation by free radicals are believed to be the main factors in the development of the plaques that narrow arteries in atherosclerosis. The authors of this paper drew attention to American research that showed that when vitamin E is added to cells grown in culture in the laboratory, it blocks the oxidation changes in LDLs. They also pointed out that the protective polyunsaturated fats are very vulnerable to attack by free radicals, which can start a chain reaction causing them, in turn, to become free radicals. This chain reaction can be prevented by vitamin E.

Although I have highlighted this paper, I would emphasize that this is but one of many hundreds of professional articles dealing with free radicals and heart disease that have been published in the medical press in recent years. Almost all of these support the view that free radicals have a highly significant part to play in causing heart disease. The most impressive evidence to date in favour of vitamin E, however, was reported in two papers in the *New England Journal of Medicine* in May 1993 by Dr M. R. Stampfer and others at Harvard Medical School. The first of these concerned vitamin E consumption and the risk of coronary artery disease in women. This trial involved 87,245 female nurses aged 34 to 59 years in none of whom heart disease or cancer had been diagnosed at the beginning of the trial in 1980. The vitamin intakes of all these women were known. The greatest variation in vitamin consumption was due to the fact that a proportion of these women were taking supplementary vitamin E. During an eight-year follow-up, 552 cases of coronary disease were diagnosed among these women with 115 deaths from coronary thrombosis. Some 437 women had non-fatal heart attacks. When those with the lowest vitamin E intake were compared with those with the highest intake, the latter were found to have a risk of heart attack of only 66%. Women who took supplementary vitamin E for two years or more had an even greater reduction in risk, to 59%. Taking E for short periods did not produce any apparent benefit in reducing the risk. So long-term supplements of vitamin E can, apparently, reduce the risk of heart attack to almost half.

The second paper was concerned with the effects of vitamin E intake on 39,910 male health professionals – doctors, dentists, vets, pharmacists, opticians, etc. This study began in 1986 and lasted for four years. All were believed to be free of heart disease or related conditions, such as high blood cholesterol and diabetes, at the beginning of the trial. Again, the intake of vitamins was known. There were 667 cases of coronary disease reported during the trial. The results were especially interesting in relation to vitamin E intake. In the men taking more than 60 mg of vitamin E daily, the risk of heart attack was reduced to 64% as compared with those taking less than 7.5 mg per day. Those who took supplements of 100 mg or more a day had a relative risk of 63% as compared with those who did not take any vitamin E supplements. This trial showed that the association between differences in dietary intake of vitamin E and heart risk was weak; it was only in those men taking the larger doses possible from supplementary vitamin E capsules that there was a substantial reduction in the risk.

Neither of these trials proved positively that it was the vitamin E that was reducing the risk. Critics have suggested that people who take vitamin E supplements are, by their nature, more health-conscious and may be leading healthier lives. This point was not lost on the authors of the trials, and they adjusted the figures to take into account the effects of such things as exercise, calorie intake, dietary fibre, obesity, smoking, alcohol intake, high blood pressure and routine aspirin-taking. When all these factors were considered, the figures still showed that there was a strong protective effect against heart attacks from vitamin E intake.

## *Free radicals and heart attacks*

A heart attack is different from angina. It is the consequence of an actual blockage of a coronary artery or one of its branches. Heart attacks are not, like angina, related to exertion but come on at any time. The pain is similar in nature to angina but is often more severe. It does not pass off on resting, but goes on and on. There is often a terrifying sense of impending death which, unfortunately, is often justified.

When a part of the heart muscle is completely deprived of its blood supply, it becomes swollen and soon dies. This will weaken the heart's action and may sometimes weaken the wall of the heart, but is not necessarily fatal. With luck the dead patch of muscle forms a strong scar and the heart continues to beat satisfactorily, although capable of less powerful action than before. Sometimes this process is repeated several times, and with each attack the heart is damaged further. In such cases, heart failure – the inability to keep the blood circulating adequately – is likely to occur.

Modern research indicates that, quite apart from the effect of free radicals in causing atherosclerosis in the coronary arteries, they have another sinister role to play in heart attacks. This research has shown that a further and most important effect of free radicals occurs, not at the time of the blockage, but when the damaged tissue, especially that around the dead zone, is trying to recover by widening nearby blood vessels. This response is called 'reperfusion' and it is during this period that more oxygen becomes available and the maximum secondary danger from free radicals occurs.

This fact was dramatically illustrated in a paper published in the *Lancet* in April 1993. Free radical research has now progressed to the stage at which evidence of the presence of free radicals can actually be obtained by analyzing a small sample of the blood emerging in a vein from the area concerned. Such blood is examined by a very advanced method known as 'electron paramagnetic resonance spectroscopy'. Samples have to be stored at very low temperatures in liquid nitrogen until they can be examined.

The paper in the *Lancet* describes the case of a 61-year-old man who was treated in hospital two and a half hours after having a heart attack. A special kind of X-ray called 'angiography' showed that one of his coronary arteries was blocked. A fine tube (catheter) with a small balloon at one end was passed into the affected artery, pushed along to the obstruction, and the balloon inflated. The artery was successfully opened up. So far, the matter was routine. This procedure of coronary artery balloon angioplasty is a day-to-day routine, too commonplace to be reported in a medical journal. What was different about this case was that, before passing the balloon catheter, a second, very narrow-bore, tube had been passed into the patient's heart so that the tip lay near the opening of the vein – the coronary sinus – that returns the coronary artery blood to the circulation. This allowed samples of the blood passing through the affected area to be taken throughout the procedure. These were immediately frozen to await spectroscopy.

Unfortunately, an hour later, the coronary artery closed again and the procedure had to be repeated. Again, samples of blood emerging from the affected area were obtained and processed. This time, the artery remained open long-term, and all was well. When the blood samples were studied by electron paramagnetic resonance spectroscopy it was found that, in both episodes, each time the artery was opened up a flood of free radicals poured out of the area.

This was an important confirmation of the widely held view that a great deal of the damage that occurs in the course of a heart attack is caused by free radicals that are released during the recovery phase, whether from the body's natural recovery response by opening up nearby blood vessels, or whether due to medical intervention. The experts currently believe that it is the increased availability of oxygen, at this point, that initiates the production of free radicals.

## *Later free radical damage*

It seems that the free radicals still have not completed their deadly work. It has been known for many years that as soon as heart muscle is damaged by loss of its blood supply, millions of scavenging white blood cells (phagocytes) move into the area to start cleaning it up so that healing and scar formation can proceed. What was not known until recently, is that this 'leucocyte infiltration', as it is known in medical jargon, is also associated with a burst of free radical production. The reason for this is that phagocytes actually use free radicals in their cleaning-up operations. In the case described here, the monitoring of free radicals was continued and, sure enough, between 9 and 24 hours after the procedure there was a rise in the output of free radicals that went even higher than when the coronary artery was opened up on the first and second occasions. Such free radical production is probably necessary, but there is a real possibility that it is also responsible for further damage to the heart. Phagocyte free radical overproduction has been investigated in several other diseases.

## *Practical implications and a warning*

Scientific medicine looks for explanations of disease processes before attempting to find cures. 'Try-it-and-see' methods – known as 'empirical treatments' – are all very well and are certainly adopted if the evidence for their efficacy is strong enough. But until there is a provable explanation of how they work, there is always a lingering doubt, and this doubt is sometimes later found to have been justified. Now that so much is known about the role of free radicals in the production of disease damage, the stage is set for attempts at intervention to try to minimize this damage. Such intervention must obviously take the form of an attack on the free radicals, either by the use of various antioxidants or by other means.

Medical interest in this possibility is now intense and many trials are being conducted. I must emphasize, however, that the basic problem in heart attacks is the narrowing and obstruction of the coronary arteries. Everything possible must be done, from the earliest stage, to minimize the risk of such narrowing or blockage. Since free radicals play an important role in causing the arterial disease that brings about this narrowing, we have one obvious line of approach. It would be totally wrong, however, on this account to deflect attention from the importance of the already established risk factors – smoking, obesity, high blood pressure, lack of exercise and a diet high in saturated fats. Free radicals are not the whole story and anyone who thinks that a regular daily dose of vitamin E and vitamin C confers a licence to continue the life of an overeating, overweight, cigarette-smoking, physically idle couch potato would be very foolish indeed.

# 4
# Antioxidants and Cancer

It would be wonderful to be able to tell you that the cancer problem has been solved by antioxidant research. Regrettably I can't. The significance of free radicals in relation to cancer is less clear than in the case of arterial and heart disease, and, sadly, no breakthrough has yet been achieved. Nevertheless, an enormous amount of research is going on to see how the risk of cancer is affected by the blood levels of the antioxidant vitamins. These studies have shown that there is a strong association between diet and cancer and have highlighted the kind of diets most likely to protect against cancer. This is a self-help matter in which knowledge and the determination to act on it can make a world of difference to us all.

The results of this research are described below.

## *What is cancer?*

The word 'cancer' is a convenient general term, used by doctors to refer to over 200 different conditions. Cancer can start up in any body tissue or organ. This is called 'primary cancer'. Or it can spread form a primary site to affect other parts of the body. Some cancers, like rodent ulcers of the skin, are so minor that they can be cured by a needle prick and ten minutes of painless surgery. Others are so malignant that long before any signs appear, the disease may already be beyond remedy and resists every attempt at treatment. The common small cell bronchial carcinoma (lung cancer), caused by cigarette smoking, is often of this type. There is, however, an important sense in which cancer is a single disease. All cancer cells, whatever their origin and type, share a common set of basic changes and follow a common pattern of abnormal behaviour. They all show very similar, or even identical, changes.

Most human body tissues are composed of millions of tiny microscopic cells. Normal tissue cells remain localized in their particular organs, growing and reproducing very slowly and just sufficiently to make up for accidental cell death. When cells are tightly packed together and unable to move, they reproduce slowly. This is called 'contact inhibition'. If the cell density is reduced, cell movement occurs and this is associated with an increased rate of reproduction. Liver cells, for instance, normally grow very slowly, no faster than is necessary to make up for wear and tear. But if a piece of liver is removed, the surrounding cells will multiply rapidly, regenerating liver tissue, until the deficiency is restored. In cancer, the normal contact inhibition does not work and cell replication is rapid and unchecked. Unlike normal cells, cancer cells also frequently move into tissue of a different type from those of their place of origin.

## *Benign and malignant tumours*

The word 'tumour' does not necessarily mean a cancer. There are two categories of tumours – benign and malignant – and the difference is important. Benign tumours are not cancers. They are just lumps of cells which, while still closely resembling the tissue from which they have arisen – muscle, nerve, fat, blood vessel, and so on – have begun to multiply more rapidly than normal. They remain intact, form a capsule, and grow by expansion only. Malignant tumours are quite different. They do not remain in a well-defined, circumscribed lump, insulated from surrounding tissue. Their nature is invasive, and they stretch out in columns which pass into nearby tissues, crossing body barriers, spreading along surfaces, seeding off into blood and lymph vessels, and usually reproducing and growing at a much faster rate than normal cells.

A cancer starting with one small group of cells has to divide many times before reaching a mass large enough to be detected. The smallest such detectable mass is of the order of 1 gram. Cancers are usually fatal when the tumour mass has reached 500 gram to 1 kg. This size is reached after only 10 further doublings of the 1 gram mass.

## *Mutations and cancer*

Malignant tumours are collections of cells which have suffered a mutation (change) in their genetic material (DNA). Most major mutations are lethal; the affected cell dies and no further harm is done. Some mutations, however, cause cells to reproduce in a wholly disorganized and uncontrolled manner, causing a cancer. All important cell functions, especially reproduction, are under the control of DNA. Damaged DNA does not, of course, necessarily cause a cell to become cancerous; but certain kinds of DNA change will disrupt normal gene regulation, activate certain tumour-producing genes known as 'oncogenes' and, in this way, induce cancer. Any agency that can damage DNA is thus potentially capable of causing cancer, and we know of a number of things – radiation, certain chemicals and viruses – that can cause these changes. Radiation and dangerous chemicals do their harm by producing free radicals, so these are clearly implicated in the stage of chemical damage to DNA.

## *How cancers spread*

Cancers spread in two ways. They burrow into and invade adjacent tissues and structures, becoming incorporated into them and often destroying them. But they have another, and even more dangerous, way of spreading. When an invading cancer encounters a small blood vessel, it can grow through the wall until it reaches the bloodstream, and small collections of cancer cells can then be carried off by the fast-flowing blood to be deposited in another part of the body. This is called 'metastasis' and is the major cause of death in cancer. By this means, cancer cells from the lung or colon or prostate gland can be transported to the brain or bones or liver, to set up a new focus and continue to grow and invade in the new site. In the absence of effective treatment, metastatic cancer is usually fatal.

Unfortunately, many people with cancers apparently confined to one site already have small inapparent metastases (micrometastases) in distant parts of the body. So even radical surgical removal of the primary tumour may not cure the cancer, which may appear in the new sites. It is for this reason that anticancer drugs, which have their effect wherever the cancer may be throughout the body, are often given in addition to surgery in cases in which such metastases are suspected.

## *Degrees of malignancy*

Cancers vary enormously in the speed with which they spread locally and, consequently, in the readiness with which they form new colonies elsewhere. This tendency is called 'malignancy' and malignancy may be low or high. A tumour of low malignancy may take many months or even years to cause trouble and may not spread distantly for a very long time, if ever.

Unfortunately, tumours of high malignancy will sometimes have spread widely before the victim has any idea that anything is wrong. Skilled pathologists can usually tell, by examining a thin slice of cancer tissue under a microscope, whether it is of high or low malignancy. In tumours of low malignancy, the cells quite closely resemble the parent tissue and form themselves into aggregates which are not greatly different in structure from the normal tissue from which they arise. Very malignant cells, on the other hand, are 'primitive', simple cells with little or no capacity to form recognizable tissues.

## *The effects of cancer*

Cancers are, of course, destructive. Some become very large and cause local effects by their sheer physical bulk – by compressing or displacing important structures. They erode and damage organs and blood vessels, block tubes, destroy vital functional tissue, form abnormal connections between organs and body cavities, promote internal bleeding and the production of abnormal quantities of fluid, and allow access to infecting organisms.

In addition, cancers have general effects. These are caused by chemical substances, often proteins, released by the tumour cells and carried throughout the body by the bloodstream. Some of these substances resemble hormones and can have widespread and severe effects. Some tumours manufacture a wide range of these hormone-like substances. The small cell cancers of the lung, for instance, can produce hormones affecting the calcification of bone, the lining of the womb, the output of the adrenal glands leading to high blood pressure and other effects, and the function of the kidneys leading to inability to excrete enough water. Breast cancers and some lung and kidney tumours can produce hormones which raise the levels of blood calcium to dangerous degrees, causing vomiting, excessive urinary output and coma.

In addition to the hormone-like effects, tumours produce a variety of general effects, not all of which are fully understood. These include nausea, loss of appetite, anaemia, fever, skin rashes, weakness, abnormalities of taste sensation, and severe and progressive loss of weight. The end result is often the severely debilitated state, with gross weight loss, known as 'cachexia', and this is often terminal. Cachexia may result from malnutrition from bowel obstruction or defective absorption of food or simply from the loss of appetite which is a common feature of widespread cancer. In addition, tumour cells have a greater demand for amino acids – the 'building bricks' of protein – than normal cells, and may use these up at the expense of the patient's muscles so that body wasting occurs.

The cause of death in people with widespread cancer is usually a combination of several factors such as cachexia, infection, internal bleeding, and compression of vital tissue – such as the brain – by a growing tumour mass. Actual destruction of essential structures is a less common cause of death.

## *Diet and cancer*

This has become an important subject and an enormous amount of research is going on to investigate it. In 1997 the World Cancer Research Fund, in association with the American Institute for Cancer Research, published a 670-page book called *Food, Nutrition and the Prevention of Cancer*. As may be expected, a book as recent as this contains a great deal of information about antioxidant vitamins. It also contains an enormous amount of detail about the effects on the incidence of various kinds of cancers of diets that are low in vegetables and fruit.

So far as vitamin C is concerned, there is now clear evidence that people with low dietary vitamin C intake – that is, people who do not eat much in the way of vegetables and fruit – are more likely to get most forms of cancer than people who eat normal amounts of C-containing food. Here is a brief summary of the diet and cancer findings derived from numerous research projects:

- the risk of cancers of the mouth and throat is decreased by diets high in fruit and vegetables;
- the risk of cancers of the larynx is lower in those with diets high in fruit and vegetables;
- the risk of cancer of the oesophagus is reduced in people whose diets are high in fruit and vegetables;
- there is convincing evidence that diets high in fruit and vegetables are protective against cancer of the lung;
- five trials of vitamin C found a significant or strongly protective effect against lung cancer;
- diets high in fruit and vegetables appear to protect against pancreatic cancer;
- diets high in vegetables decrease the risk of colon and rectal cancer;
- diets high in vegetables and fruit probably decrease the risk of breast cancer;
- the most effective dietary way of avoiding cancers of the ovary and the lining of the womb is to ensure a high intake of fruit and vegetables;
- diets high in vegetables and low in animal fats offer some protection against prostate cancer;
- diets high in vegetables and fruit probably protect against bladder cancer;
- there is, as yet, no convincing evidence that dietary factors can affect cervical cancer.

So far as trials of antioxidant vitamin supplements are concerned, the evidence is, until now, scanty. Unfortunately, most of the trials of supplements have used combinations, many including beta-carotene, and we now know that beta-carotene supplements cause more harm than good. Some research, however, came up with encouraging results. In one trial, daily supplements of 50 mg of vitamin E was associated with a 34% reduction in the incidence of prostate cancer, but had no effect on lung cancer. An Italian trial of supplementary vitamins C and E showed a significant reduction in precancerous polyps of the colon in predisposed people. Other trials showed no protective effect in this condition (familial polyposis). The precancerous mouth condition of leukoplakia was caused wholly or partially to disappear in 65% of people who were given vitamin E supplements of 400 mg twice a day for 24 weeks. A large study of women's health involving 40,000 American women includes vitamin E supplements, but this has not yet been completed.

As a result of all this research, it is now generally accepted by the experts that the incidence of many of the cancers which afflict Western societies could be reduced by modifying our diet. Much of this evidence comes from observing differences in the number of cases of various cancers in populations with different eating habits.

Quite apart from antioxidant vitamins, Western diets contain a staggeringly large number of different ingredients, and to the basic foodstuffs are added a legion of additional substances – condiments, flavouring agents, flavour enhancers, sweeteners, preservatives, colouring agents, emulsifiers, solvents, antioxidants, stabilizers, bulking agents, antifoaming agents and others. All of these are, of course, tested for safety, but their very number, and the possibility that some might act on others with harmful effect, impose a major problem for the government agencies concerned.

At present, only a few substances known to be capable of causing cancer have been identified as possible dietary elements. Such substances are known as 'carcinogens'. An example of these is aflatoxin, a poison produced by the common food contaminant mould *Aspergillus flavus*. *Aspergillus* grows readily on damp grains and nuts and is a common contaminant of peanuts. It is believed to cause many thousands of cases of primary liver cancer each year in countries in which food is stored in unsatisfactory conditions. Most cases occur in people whose livers have already been damaged by hepatitis B.

Other known cancer-causing substances include:

- nitrosamines, produced by overcooking or smoking of animal protein, but not yet positively identified as a cause of cancer in humans;
- nitrates and nitrite preservatives, which may form nitrosamines from dietary protein;
- salt fish, widely eaten in the Far East, and believed to be related to the development of cancer of the back of the nose;

- bracken fern, which is known to cause cancer in animals, and is popular in Japanese diets and thought to be associated with cancer of the gullet.

Less certain are the suggestions that stomach cancer is caused by highly spiced food; highly acidic foodstuffs such as pickles; nitrates in water; and irritants such as the concentrated alcohol in spirits. There is good evidence that mouth and stomach cancers are higher in heavy drinkers than in moderate or non-drinkers.

We know that a high fat diet can cause cancer in animals. The United States National Research Council, in their 1982 report, *Diet, Nutrition and Cancer*, judged that the evidence linking dietary fat and cancer in humans was stronger than for any other dietary constituent. They recommended, on these grounds alone, that the public should reduce fat intake, both saturated and unsaturated. The evidence consists mainly of the strong link, in various countries, between the number of cases of cancer, especially of the breast and colon, and the consumption of fat. The number of cases has increased proportionately with an increase in the fat intake and has also increased in immigrants to countries with a higher fat intake than the countries of origin. Remember, however, that a high fat intake nearly always implies a low fibre intake and it is possible that the effect may be caused by low dietary fibre rather than high dietary fat. The evidence linking high fibre diets and a low incidence of cancer and other bowel diseases is very strong and is generally accepted.

## *Worldwide research*

It is good to be able to report that, apart from the huge amount of general cancer research in progress – which has already made substantial advances into our understanding of the subject – a great deal of research specifically into the question of free radicals and cancer is under way. Many trials, sponsored by the American Institute for Cancer Research, are in progress to discover the role of dietary factors, including vitamins C and E, in the development of cancer. In Britain, too, much research is in progress. The Imperial Cancer Research Fund, the Medical Research Council, the Dunn Nutrition Unit and the Department of Community Medicine at Cambridge University, among many other authorities, are engaged in long-term studies, involving thousands of subjects, into the effects of dietary elements on the incidence of cancer. Huge similar projects are also under way in France, Germany, Spain, Italy, Denmark, Sweden, the Netherlands and Greece.

## *Preliminary findings*

Reports, to date, suggest that vitamins C and E and beta-carotene do offer protection against certain cancers, such as those of the lungs, oesophagus (gullet), stomach and large intestine. In particular, vitamin C is believed by some experts to be the body's major protective element against stomach cancer. This, if true, is especially important because stomach cancer is one of the most dangerous and least easily detected kinds, and is often fatally advanced before it is diagnosed.

We are still a long way from fully understanding the role of free radicals in the development of cancer. We do not even know whether their contribution is major or minor. There are, however, some very suggestive points in the story and since many cancers are so frightful and the antioxidants vitamins C and E are so safe, it is perhaps not surprising that many of the researchers engaged in this work are, like myself, taking their regular daily megadoses of these vitamins.

# 5
# Antioxidants and Ageing

Contrary to what most people think, the human life span is not steadily increasing. People are certainly living longer but only because they are getting nearer to, or reaching, the normal upper age limit of about 100 years. Life expectancy is increasing because medical and technological advances are enabling an increasing proportion of people to avoid death before reaching the full span. Today, in Western societies, for the first time in history, most people can look forward, with reasonable confidence, to growing old.

## *What puts the limit on our life span?*

Like most human characteristics, ageing is determined by the interaction of genetic and environmental factors. By 'environmental factors' I mean everything caused by the external world that can happen to a person from the moment of conception. No one knows for sure whether genes or the environment is the more important but we do know that both matter a great deal. There is not much we can do about our genes but we are certainly in a position to do something about our environment. And, as we have already seen, one of the important environmental factors is diet.

The human body is a machine that can keep itself going for 100 years. To do this, it must constantly effect running repairs by replacing cells and tissues that have been damaged or killed. This process of cell replication is going on all the time in our bodies at different rates in different cell types. Those in the reproductive organs, and those subject to most wear and tear (such as those of the skin or the lining of the bowel) require the most frequent division. You may be surprised to learn that there is a limit to the number of times cells can replace themselves.

## *Growing cells in the laboratory*

It is a fairly easy matter to investigate, in the laboratory, the number of times cell replacement cycles can occur. Growing cell cultures artifically in glass dishes (*in vitro*) is now routine. We can arrange suitable nutrition and growing surfaces for cells, so that they can survive and reproduce themselves outside the body.

When normal body cells are cultured, it is found that they will never reproduce more often than a certain number of times. Different types of cells have to reproduce a different number of times, but for each type the number is remarkably constant. Cells called 'fibroblasts' from a fetus or young baby will double in number between forty and sixty times and the culture will then die out. But if cells are taken from a middle-aged man and cultured, the number of doublings before the cells die will be reduced to about twenty-five. Cells from a very old person may not reproduce at all.

It seems that the limiting factor is not the age of the culture but solely the number of times the cells reproduce. Even keeping the cells in suspended animation by freezing for several years does not alter this fact. They will just resume where they left off, undergo the unchanging fifty or so doublings, then die. Cells from a wide range of human donors, of ages from birth to ninety years, show a steady average decrease in the number of times they reproduce before the culture dies.

## *Shortening chromosomes*

The reason for this finite number of doublings became apparent when Dr Calvin Harley, a biochemist at McMaster University, Hamilton, Ontario discovered that older cells had shorter chromosomes than younger cells. To prevent loss of vital genetic material, the ends of chromosomes are made of apparently unimportant 'junk' DNA that carries no genes and can be lost without ill effect. These end segments are called 'telomeres'. With each cell division, some of this junk DNA is shaved off. Eventually, the whole telomere is lost so that some of the true genetic material is exposed and removed. When this happens the affected cells become irretrievably damaged. When the telomeres are lost, chromosomes, being 'bare-ended', sometimes stick together at the ends, thus interfering with cell division.

Unfortunately, cancer cells have an enzyme called 'telomerase' that enables them to preserve their telomeres so they can go on dividing indefinitely. Cultured cancer cells can be immortal. A great deal of excitement was aroused at the beginning of 1998 when it was announced that telomerase could be used to allow cells that had reached the end of their 'natural' life to go on dividing.

The limit on cell reproduction is not, of course, the only factor that causes ageing. More than a hundred different changes in the structure and function of cells have been noted to occur, long before they lose the ability to replicate. These changes, which increase progressively as the number of cell divisions is used up, progressively impair the cell's ability to perform its proper functions. It is these changes which produce all the well-known signs of old age and which result in the death of the individual, around the age of one hundred years, even before the cells cease to divide.

## *Free radicals and ageing*

The basis of the free radical theory of ageing is the suggestion that free radicals are more readily and plentifully formed in older people. We know that free radicals can damage any tissue in the body. The outer membranes of cells, which contain fatty material such as cholesterol, are especially susceptible to damage by oxidation by free radicals. Such increased free radical production and damage might result from the cumulative effect of environmental influences, or from a reduction in the availability of body antioxidants, possibly from an age-related diminution in the activity of natural antioxidants.

We have seen how widespread and seriously damaging are the effects of the arterial disease, atherosclerosis (see p. 29). This disease obviously contributes importantly to the bodily changes characteristic of ageing. And we have also seen how important is free radical oxidation of low-density lipoproteins in the development of atherosclerosis. So far as diseases are concerned, atherosclerosis is by far the most important cause of shortening of life. Statistically, it is far more important than cancer.

The third link between free radicals and ageing is the effect on

DNA. Not all the DNA occurs in the chromosomes. All cells contain thousands of tiny energy-producing bodies known as 'mitochondria' and these, too, contain a genome of DNA. Interestingly, the mitochondrial DNA comes in the non-nuclear part of the cell and so is derived from the egg, not the sperm. It is thus inherited only from the mother. Mitochondrial DNA is now known to be especially vulnerable to free radical damage, possibly because it is so concerned with oxidative chemical reactions. Any unrepaired free radical damage to this DNA would have a serious effect on the continued functioning of the cell. Scientists estimate that oxygen free radicals cause thousands of DNA base changes (mutations) every day, the great majority of which are automatically repaired. But even the most efficient repair mechanism is unlikely to pick up and correct every mutation.

## *The role of antioxidants*

It is now well established that there is a positive correlation between diet and length of life. In many animal species, lifespan can be increased up to 50% by suitable modification of the diet. Whether this enhancement is due to a reduction in free radical action, so that bodily antioxidants can more readily cope, remains to be seen. There is evidence that rats on low-calorie diets suffer less free radical damage to their body proteins than those on unrestricted diets. This may be because they have larger quantities of the important enzymes that protect against free radicals (see p. 25). But antioxidants are unlikely to be the whole story, for in rats living longer on restricted diets there is known to be increased expression of certain genes in liver tissue. So genetic factors are also probably involved.

There is, however, some more direct evidence of increased free radical action with age. Scientists at the University of Kentucky have been studying the performance of gerbils in running mazes. Old gerbils, on average, make twice as many mistakes as young gerbils. But if old gerbils are given the free radical-trapping antioxidant, butyl-alpha-phenylnitrone (PBN) for two weeks, their performance improves so as to be every bit as good as that of young gerbils. When the PBN is stopped, they go back to making as many mistakes as before.

The researcher, Thomas Johnson, of the University of Colorado has been able to breed a strain of roundworm with a lifespan more than twice that of others of the same species. The remarkable thing about these long-living worms is that they have significantly higher levels of the enzymes superoxide dismutase and catalase (see p. 25) than their less fortunate friends. These enzymes are natural antioxidants and are exactly the same as those that protect humans against free radicals.

It is, of course, arguable whether one can safely apply to humans results that have been obtained on little white furry rodents and roundworms. But the findings in these animal experiments do make it clear that, in a range of living creatures, there is an important link between antioxidants and ageing.

Here is another piece of strongly suggestive evidence. Proteins that have been damaged by free radical oxidation can be detected by highly sensitive tests for particular bits of protein components (amino acids) that are released in the course of the damage. Post-mortem examinations on human brains show that old people have more of these bits in their brains than do young people. The inference is that natural antioxidants are not working as well in older people as they do in the young. If this is so, there is a strong probability that supplementary antioxidant vitamins can make up for the age-related deficiencies of the natural antioxidants that mop up free radicals in younger people.

## *The opinions of scientists*

As long ago as 1956, the research scientist D. Harmon, writing in a medical journal devoted to the science of ageing, the *Journal of Gerontology*, suggested that free radicals are probably involved in the ageing process. Since then the free radical theory of ageing has become widely accepted. Gerontologists now generally believe that free radical damage to tissues is a central factor in the development of most of the age-related diseases – atherosclerosis, arthritis, loss of muscle and heart efficiency, cataract, rheumatoid arthritis, lung disorders, skin deterioration and probably cancer.

Earl R. Stadtman, Chief of the Biochemistry Laboratory at the National Heart, Lung, and Blood Institute, National Institutes of Health, Bethesda, Maryland, writing in *Science* – the American equivalent of the British *Nature* – in August 1992, summarized the current scientific views on free radical oxidation of proteins and ageing. He confirmed the general opinion that free radicals are responsible for much damage to cell membranes and DNA, and described in detail the way proteins – the essential building materials of the body – are attacked by hydroxyl radicals (see p. 21) produced by radiation and ozone, and by hydroxyl and other radicals produced in the body. The evidence he quotes suggests that anything up to 50% of the cellular protein in old people might be present in the damaged oxidized form.

This hard-headed scientist ends the paper with the carefully restrained statement: 'There is reason for hope that a pharmacological intervention may be found to ameliorate age-related disorders.' In other words, we have reason to believe that it may become possible to reduce many of the effects of ageing by taking antioxidant vitamins.

# 6
# Cut the Risk of Cataract

One of the most striking features of the medical literature on free radicals and antioxidants is the ever-increasing number of medical conditions that are being shown to be affected. So far, the visual system has received comparatively little attention, but interest is growing and it seems probable that, before long, many eye disorders will be seen to be mediated by free radical damage. One major eye disorder which affects millions of people and causes great distress has, however, prompted a number of very interesting and productive research projects. That condition is cataract.

## *Cataract*

Many people are slightly confused about cataract and think it involves the outer lens of the eye – the cornea. Others have the idea that it is a 'skin' growing over some part of the eye. Both notions are wrong. The misunderstanding is partly due to advertisements for charities asking for money to support cataract surgery teams in the Third World. These are highly deserving charities that do excellent work, but their publicity is liable to show well-meaning but misleading photographs of people with dense, white corneal scars – which are not cataracts.

Cataract is simply a loss of transparency of the internal focusing lens of the eye – the 'crystalline' lens that lies immediately behind the coloured iris and that can be seen only through the pupil. The name arose centuries ago from the fanciful idea that the whiteness in the pupil – which, incidentally, is seen only in long-neglected cases – was a kind of waterfall descending from the brain. In a dense cataract, the pupil may indeed appear white but the appearance is due to aggregation of the lens proteins known as 'crystallins' – changes rather like those that occur in the transparent albumen of an egg when it is boiled.

Even the most dense cataract never entirely eliminates perception of light so, although cataract can fog out any useful image, it never causes complete blindness in the sense that nothing is seen at all. An eye that can perceive no light at all has something more seriously wrong with it than simply cataract. Often the opacity involves only the rear part of the lens, and so a person may have a severe defect of vision while still having a perfectly normal-looking eye.

## *Causes of cataract*

Although cataracts can be caused by virus infection before birth, penetrating or blunt injury, severe diabetes, Down's syndrome and various other things, the great majority of cataracts occur, apparently spontaneously, as an age-related effect in elderly people. Most people over about 75 years have some detectable loss of visual clarity from cataract. Many have a marked degree of visual deterioration but, because the effects of age-related cataract on vision come on so gradually and adaptation is so good, a great many people with quite severe opacities will deny that there is anything wrong.

Eventually, however, many find that they cannot drive cars, read or even watch TV with any satisfaction. Unfortunately, many people in this situation accept their disability as a 'normal' feature of ageing and do nothing about it. This is a great pity as the results of cataract surgery, with intra-ocular lens implantation – assuming there is nothing else wrong with the eye – are excellent, and cataract operations are among the most successful of all surgical procedures. Indeed, the condition is so remediable that ophthalmic surgeons faced with patients suffering from severe loss of vision are usually mentally hoping that the trouble is cataract. In spite of this, the prospect of surgery on the eyes is usually daunting, sometimes frightening, to the patient.

## *Symptoms of cataract*

Cataract cannot cause pain and never does. Its only effect is on the quality of vision. The condition comes on almost imperceptibly and nearly always progresses very slowly. Usually the progress of the opacification is steady, but sometimes there are brief accelerations and then longer periods when little change is apparent. Many cataracts alter the way in which different light wavelengths pass through the lens, so that red and yellow light can pass through more easily than blue light. Again, the effect is gradual and may not be readily noticeable, but after cataract surgery it is commonplace for patients to exclaim with pleasure at the unaccustomed brightness of the sky or of blue objects.

Another effect of increased density in the lens is to increase its power of bending light rays. This is known as an increase in the refractive index of the lens. The effect is that the person affected may become gradually more and more short-sighted. This often allows them, at least for a time, to read without reading glasses, and may even promote the illusion that the vision is improving. The ability to make out near detail is, however, always accompanied by blurring of distant objects. People in this situation sometimes buy a succession of ever-stronger glasses for distance vision and spend a lot of money in an eventually hopeless quest for visual clarity. There is no harm in this, except to the bank balance.

The most important symptom of cataract is progressive loss of visual clarity in the centre of the field of vision. This is very annoying and disabling, especially if the lens opacities cause scattering of the light. Some people first become aware that something is wrong when they find they have to give up driving at night because of the dangerously blinding glare from the headlights of approaching cars. Many, on the other hand, are quite unaware of such effects and simply recognize that they cannot see so well as they used to. Once the lens protein has become denatured and the fibres disorganized, there is no possible way to restore transparency. The only remedy is to remove the opaque lens completely and replace it with a tiny, optically perfect plastic lens implant of a power calculated to focus the eye correctly.

## *Cataract and free radicals*

The mechanisms of the development of age-related cataract are still a matter of argument, but it is becoming increasingly obvious that oxidation (see p. 22) of the lens protein is an important factor. The fine protein fibres of which the internal lenses are made are themselves transparent. The transparency of the lens as a whole depends on the uniformity of diameter of these fibres and the evenness and parallelism with which they are laid down in the lens. When protein is damaged, this uniformity of structure is lost, and the fibres, instead of transmitting light evenly, cause it to be scattered and even reflected. The result is severely defective vision.

The view that age-related cataract may be due to free radical damage is indirect but very strong and is based largely on the differences between the levels of antioxidants (see p. 24) in the bodies of people with cataract compared with those in comparable people with clear lenses. These trials have been reported in various respectable medical and scientific journals such as the *British Medical Journal*, *Archives of Ophthalmology*, *Annals of the New York Academy of Science*, and the *American Journal of Clinical Nutrition*.

One of the most impressive studies was carried out in the Department of Biomedical Sciences, University of Tampere, Finland, and published in the *British Medical Journal* in December 1992. In this project, 47 people with cataract and a carefully selected comparable group of 94 people with clear lenses were compared. The normal 'controls' were selected to be as similar as possible to those with cataracts in terms of age, sex, occupation, smoking history, blood cholesterol levels, body weight, blood pressure and the presence or absence of diabetes. All had blood samples taken that were analysed by highly sensitive methods for levels of vitamin E and beta-carotene. Beta-carotene is the orange pigment in carrots and other vegetables that is converted in the liver to vitamin A.

The results showed that there was a significant relationship between the levels of vitamin E and beta-carotene and the likelihood of having cataract. Low blood levels of these antioxidant vitamins were found in the cataract group; higher levels in the clear lens controls. People low in both vitamins were two and a half times as likely to have cataracts as those with higher levels. The authors of the study concluded: 'Low serum concentrations of the antioxidant vitamins alpha-tocopherol (vitamin E) and beta-carotene are risk factors for end stage senile cataract.

Controlled trials of the role of antioxidant vitamins in cataract prevention are therefore warranted.'

Another study, carried out in Canada and reported at an international conference, involved 175 cataract patients and the same number of people with clear lenses. Again, this study showed a meaningful difference in the intake of vitamins E and C in the two groups. Those who had taken extra C and E vitamins for five years or more were significantly more numerous in the clear lens group than in the cataract group. The epidemiologist, Professor James Robertson, head of the project, said, 'Supplementary vitamins C and E are associated with a significant reduction in risk of cataracts.'

## *Free radicals and ultraviolet light*

Many scientists now suspect that at least one source of cataract-producing free radicals is ultraviolet light – which is present in large quantity in sunlight. Some have even suggested that this is the reason why cataracts occur much earlier in countries such as India than in more temperate areas. It is already well established that ultraviolet radiation produces free radicals in tissue. Ultraviolet light is the cause of sunburning and of the age-related damage to skin found in people with a history of long exposure to sunlight (see p. 64.). These are free radical effects. It is also the cause of much external eye irritation and of the condition of pterygium in which a fold of the membrane covering the white of the eye (the conjunctiva) moves across over the cornea. Surface eye tissues, being transparent, are very susceptible to ultraviolet light and, in view of recent developments, it seems almost certain that these changes are induced by free radicals.

Because the internal lens of the eye is protected by the cornea and by a layer of water behind the cornea, both of which partially absorb ultraviolet light, ophthalmologists have been less ready to accept that ultraviolet light is an important cause of cataract. In recent years, however, this view has gained increasing support. The idea that free radicals are involved is supported by research conducted at the University of Maryland by the biochemist, Professor Shambu Varma. Isolated lenses exposed to strong light stresses became cloudy, but this could be prevented if the solution in which the lenses were placed contained antioxidants. Professor Varma also recommended that people should take supplementary vitamins C and E, at least from around the age of 40, to protect the lenses against later cataract formation.

## *Smoking and cataract*

There is an important link between cataract and smoking that should be of interest to everyone. Separate studies of smoking and the incidence of cataract in men and women, published in the *Journal of the American Medical Association* in August 1992, have shown that people who smoke 20 or more cigarettes a day are about twice as likely to develop cataract as non-smokers. The men concerned were 22,071 American doctors and the women were 50,828 American registered nurses.

The explanation of this has to be related to the lower concentrations of the antioxidant vitamins C and E in the blood of smokers. Lens damage in cataract is oxidative damage of the lens protein. Cigarette smoke is rich in free radicals and other oxidative substances such as aldehydes. We know that free radicals from cigarette smoke can damage proteins. In view of all this it is hardly surprising that smokers are more prone to cataract than non-smokers.

Whatever you do, don't let this information persuade you that smoking can be made safer by taking antioxidant vitamins. All smokers are very good at latching on to any convenient rationalization to allow them to continue. This one would be particularly dangerous. In my professional experience I have seen far too many tragedies, far too many promising lives cut short, far too many people turned into respiratory and cardiac cripples to be able to contemplate smoking with equanimity. We are now beginning to understand in much more detail how smoking damages the body and this understanding includes details of a great many processes that have nothing to do with free radicals.

## *Free radicals and the premature eye*

Very small babies must often be nursed in atmospheres of oxygen in incubators if their lives are to be preserved. Unfortunately, all eye specialists have become familiar with the devastating effects of excessive oxygen on the eyes of these premature infants. Too much oxygen produces free radicals, and the immature tissues of the infants are especially vulnerable to their damaging effects. There is severe damage to the retina and an abnormal budding-out of fronds and tangles of new blood vessels that produce a white mass behind the lens, known as 'retrolental fibroplasia', which can completely obscure vision. Detachment of the retina may also occur, as may high degrees of short sight (myopia).

These tragic results have been seen only too often in the past in very small babies who have had to be incubated. Happily, now that doctors are alive to the risk and are carefully monitoring the amount of oxygen given, severe cases are much less common. Today, the effects are usually limited to scarring and distortion of the retinas and, of course, vary widely. In one study of 572 infants of birth weight below 1,700 grams, half had visible signs of the disorder. Happily, the great majority of these cleared up without treatment. As might be expected, the lower the birth weight and the shorter the pregnancy, the greater the severity. Paediatricians often have to make agonizing decisions in which they must balance the risk to the life of the baby against the risk to its vision.

The premature eye is vulnerable because it already has a plentiful oxygen supply and an unusually high rate of oxidation. It also has a much higher than average number of mitochondria (see p. 122). Newborn babies have reduced blood levels of vitamin E. This typically rises to normal within two or three weeks, but in the case of premature infants this takes much longer. Such babies, therefore, have less antioxidant protection than they need.

It has, therefore, been very tempting to treat premature babies with vitamin E supplements. Here, great caution is needed. Not all free radicals are antagonistic to the body. Free radicals are the means by which certain cells of the immune system – the phagocytes – kill bacteria and viruses. It is comparatively easy in very small babies to reach very high levels of vitamin E in the blood and this may interfere with the necessary action against germs. The normal adult blood concentration of vitamin E is about 0.8 mg in every 100 cc (100 ml). Some babies treated with vitamin E have had concentrations of as high as 5 mg per 100 cc, and an increased incidence of a serious bowel infection occurred in babies on such dosage. For this reason, although some trials have shown a significant decrease in free radical eye problems, the use of vitamin E in premature infants remains highly controversial.

What this research does indicate, however, is that vitamin E is a powerful substance that can have major effects in the body and that it should be treated with respect. People often operate on the principle that you can't have too much of a good thing. As we have seen, this principle certainly does not apply in the context of self-treatment with some of the vitamins. There is no reason to suppose that reasonable doses of vitamin E are likely to cause any harm to children and adults. Excess of vitamins A and D can certainly be harmful (see p.13). Vitamin C appears to be remarkably safe.

The evidence for the protective value of vitamins C and E against cataract is very persuasive. Maybe this is yet another good reason why you should consider taking them, especially if you have reached the prime of life.

# 7

# Other Free Radical Effects and How to Minimize Them

This chapter deals with a number of seemingly unconnected conditions. But there is a common theme. All are disorders in which free radicals have been found to play an important part. One of these conditions – skin ageing – is of special interest, as it was one of the first in which it was shown possible to reverse, at least to a degree, free radical damage. This chapter also covers some little-known facts about the scavenging cells of the body – the phagocytes – and a brief glimpse at the intriguing theory that red wine may be good for you.

## *Skin ageing and free radicals*

Doctors have known for years that sunlight damages the skin. This was not especially clever as the evidence has been around for centuries. If you compare the skins of white people living mainly indoors with those of people who spend their days in the open, especially in tropical and subtropical areas, you will see that, while the former remain smooth and elastic, the latter become wrinkled, discoloured and lax. Many sun-loving people of European or American origin who live in hot areas suffer devastating skin damage, with drooping, sagging folds, extensive fine wrinkling, and a much higher than average incidence of the three common skin cancers: rodent ulcer (basal cell carcinoma), squamous cancer (squamous epithelioma) and malignant melanoma.

The scientists have known for decades that this damage is caused by ultraviolet radiation from the sun. The most obvious effect of this radiation is on the elastic collagen protein of the skin which becomes reduced in quantity and altered in quality. The result is sagging and wrinkling and loss of support to the small blood vessels of the skin. The result is what is inaccurately called 'broken veins' or telangiectasia – widening and conspicuous prominence of vessels that are normally too small to be seen. Skin specialists, recognizing that these changes are the result of light damage over long periods, call them photo-ageing.

## *Tretinoin and ageing skin*

The new knowledge concerns the way that ultraviolet radiation actually causes the damage. Paradoxically, in this case, the treatment came before the explanation. Back in 1986, a paper appeared in the *Journal of the American Academy of Dermatology* entitled, 'Topical tretinoin for photo-aged skin'. This paper recounted how the proportion of sun-damaged to normal skin collagen could be markedly reduced by treatment with the drug tretinoin. This was followed by similar papers in other journals including one in the *Journal of the American Medical Association* entitled, 'At last, a medical treatment for skin aging'. Some trials involved large numbers of patients treated with tretinoin over a period of several months. Tretinoin is all-trans-retinoic acid and is the active form of vitamin A in all the tissues of the body except the retina. It is a powerful antioxidant (see p. 24) and is sold in Britain in a 0.05% cream under the trade name of Retinova. Note that taking tretinion is not the same as taking vitamin A.

We now know, of course, that ultraviolet light causes production of free radicals and that it is these that do the damage. By the time this became clear, dermatologists already knew that they could partially reverse the effects of solar radiation on the skin by using tretinoin. In a typical trial of this treatment, one side of the face of volunteers was treated with 0.05% tretinoin cream once a day and the other side treated with the cream base without the tretinoin. At the end of 12 weeks, skin thickness, as measured by ultrasound and other methods, had increased by 10% in the areas treated with tretinoin.

Other trials of longer periods of treatment showed improvement in skin thickness, in the roughness of the skin and in fine wrinkling, but, as might be expected since much damage had already been done, did not affect sagging, age freckles (lentigines) or broken veins. The thickening of the outer skin layer, the epidermis, was, in many cases, remarkable, and could be as great as two and three-quarter times. Almost all the people in the trial suffered some degree of minor inflammation with itching and a feeling of tightness. This side effect settled on stopping the cream applications for a day or two and the treatment could then be safely resumed. These trials make it clear that people whose skin has already been severely damaged by the sun are likely to derive much less benefit from tretinoin treatment than people who have had less exposure to solar radiation. Tretinoin, under the trade name of Retin-A, is also widely used in the treatment of the adolescent skin disease acne, in which it is highly effective. It has been used by well over a million people.

## *Risk from tretinoin*

The manufacturers repeatedly warned that this drug, which has also been given by mouth, was capable of producing birth defects or even the death of the fetus, and stated that it should not be taken by women during pregnancy. Even so, a number of cases of congenital malformation were reported in fetuses born to women using the drug. There was, of course, no positive way of knowing whether these were due to the tretinoin. Congenital malformations and spontaneous abortions were also occurring in women who were not taking or using tretinoin. Reports, in the popular press, of very large numbers of cases of malformations were almost certainly exaggerated. Interestingly, a study reported in the *Lancet*, in May 1993 showed that the number of major fetal abnormalities occurring in the case of pregnant women using tretinoin preparations on the skin was the same as the number in the case of women not using the drug.

Today, tretinoin is used externally only, except for the preparation Vesanoid, which is used with other drugs in the treatment of one form of leukaemia.

## *Malignant melanoma*

In the last 50 years or so, there has been a dramatic increase in the number of cases of the highly dangerous skin tumour, malignant melanoma. There is now some evidence that antioxidant treatment with tretinoin can reduce this risk. Trials have suggested that the vitamin can normalize the early changes in the pigment cells (the melanocytes) that can progress to melanoma. They also suggest that tretinoin can retard the growth of melanomas and reduce their tendency to spread remotely. This research is still in an early stage.

If there is one lesson to be learned from all this, it is that prevention is better than cure. Sunbathing is a very bad habit. If you must do it, you should be quite sure that your skin is adequately protected by an effective sunscreen preparation.

## *Smoking and free radicals*

Smoking is by far the most dangerous use of an addictive substance. For every lung cancer death caused by smoking, there are three deaths from other smoking-related diseases. Smoking is still the largest single cause of premature death. Although large numbers of people have now been able to give up, and smoking has become a divisive social issue, there are still many who seem unable to conquer this addiction. This is not helped by the determination of the tobacco manufacturers to continue to advertise their pernicious wares – that is, to try to persuade as many people as possible to kill themselves.

Smoking wastes money, causes bad breath, body odour and stained fingers, and systematically damages many of the systems of the body so that, even if the worst doesn't happen, the long term quality of life is likely to be substantially reduced. Recent research into the relationship between free radicals and the damaging effect of smoking may, I hope, provide some smokers with better motivation to cease this hazardous practice.

## *Seminal fluid antioxidants*

Few people seem to realize that the adverse effects of smoking extend even beyond the smoker and others forced to breathe the smoker's exhalations. Epidemiologists at the University of North Carolina carried out a study of 15,000 children born between 1959 and 1966. This showed that the children of men who, prior to the birth, had smoked more than 20 cigarettes a day were twice as likely to suffer from certain genetic defects such as cleft lip and palate and congenital heart disorders. Another associated study by scientists at the National Institute of Environmental Health at North Carolina found that leukaemia and lymph node cancer were twice as common in the children of male smokers as in the children of non-smokers. Brain tumours were also significantly more common.

Interestingly, the effect seems to be on sperm DNA but not on egg (ovum) DNA. No genetic links have been found that can be attributed to smoking by the mother. This is probably because cells forming sperms are far more often in a state of division (mitosis) than are eggs. Mutations occur mostly during mitosis because repair activity is temporarily halted during this phase.

You may be wondering what all this has to do with antioxidant vitamins. Reporting these findings at an international conference on environmental causes of cancer in February 1993, the American biochemist Bruce Ames, of the University of California at Berkeley, pointed out that much of the damage resulting from smoking comes from strongly oxidizing compounds in cigarette smoke, such as free radicals. When this damage affects the DNA in the cells that produce sperms, then some of the sperms will carry mutant DNA. If a child happens to be produced by fertilization by such a damaged sperm, congenital defects will result and the resulting mutations can, as Ames put it, cause 'an effect that will reverberate down the generations'.

Ames points out that there is about eight times as much vitamin C in seminal fluid as there is in blood. This cannot be a mere coincidence. This antioxidant vitamin must play an important role in protecting sperms from genetic damage so as to minimize the number of inheritable disorders caused by mutations. Since, like all cells in the body, sperms are attacked by about 10,000 oxidizing reactions every day, they clearly need such protection. The amount of vitamin C in the seminal fluid sensitively reflects the amount present in the diet. Even more significant, a low dietary intake of vitamin C immediately produces a substantial increase in the amount of a substance called 8-hydroxydeoxyguanosine. This is a breakdown product of DNA that is produced in increased quantity when DNA is being damaged. The current official recommended daily allowance of about 60 mg is too low to produce enough vitamin C in semen to reduce this DNA damage to safe levels. Research suggests that a minimum daily intake of 250 mg should suffice. Smoking uses up much of the vitamin C levels in the body to cope with the large amounts of oxidizing compounds in absorbed smoke, so smokers are clearly at greater risk.

## *What's in cigarette smoke*

Cigarette smoke contains a very nasty mix of free radicals, and some of the thousands of substances present in inhaled smoke and absorbed into the body during smoking, can also produce free radicals. Free radicals bring about many, if not most, of the serious bodily effects associated with smoking, especially the damaging effects on the arteries. Dr Hermann Esterbauer, of the University of Graz, Austria, a prominent researcher into the biological effects of free radicals, points out that smoking, a long-recognized risk factor for heart attacks, leads to low-density lipoprotein (LDL) free radical oxidation (see p. 32), probably from the extra free radicals produced in the body by absorbed smoke ingredients. As we have seen, this is how cholesterol gets deposited in the artery walls, especially in the coronary arteries of the heart.

There is also growing speculation that the cancer risk in smoking may be largely due to free radicals. This speculation is based on some quite strong evidence. Although free radicals are hard to detect directly there are various indirect ways of determining that they have been busy. Protein breakdown products of oxidation can be detected and so can indicators of DNA oxidation damage. When DNA is damaged, it immediately tries to repair itself. This repair work is done by enzymes called 'exonucleases'. When these enzymes get to work they release the compound 8-hydroxydeoxyguanosine. This gets into the blood and is excreted in the urine.

In the December 1992 issue of the scientific journal, *Carcinogenesis*, which is dedicated to research into the causes of cancer, there is a paper from research scientists at the University of Copenhagen, Århus University and the Danish Cancer Registry.

This paper reports the results of a trial in which the quantities of this tell-tale compound in the urine of smokers is compared with the quantities in non-smokers' urine. The figures speak for themselves. The smokers' urine contained 50% more 8-hydroxy-deoxyguanosine than that of non-smokers. This means that smokers' DNA is suffering a considerably greater rate of damage than that of non-smokers.

This additional damage could be coming either from the free radicals present in cigarette smoke or from free radicals produced in the body. We know that smokers have a higher metabolic rate (the rate of build-up and break-down of body biochemicals) than non-smokers – typically 10% to 15% higher. Raised metabolic rate accelerates all kinds of biochemical reaction pathways and some of these produce free radicals.

It would be quite wrong to leave you with the impression that researchers believe that free radicals are the most important cause of smoking-induced cancer. There is plenty of evidence that other mechanisms are also at work, especially the effects of the binding to DNA of certain aromatic hydrocarbons found in cigarette smoke. Nevertheless, the current interest in the role of free radicals in this context is intense.

The tell-tale indicator of DNA damage in the urine of smokers makes them particularly suitable subjects for investigating whether the antioxidant vitamins C and E can reduce the risk of cancer. Many workers in the field now believe that the time has come for long-term trials of antioxidants. There is, however, one major difficulty. These scientists know better than most what smoking can do to the human body. They therefore have serious ethical reservations about any advance that might encourage smokers to continue. The way to avoid smoking-related body damage is to stop smoking. The scientists are at pains to point out that work of this kind is not done in the hope of trying to make smoking safer.

In addition to the monitoring of urine for 8-hydroxydeoxyguanosine, there are other ways of detecting rates of free radical damage to DNA. Lung cancer is not really cancer of the lung substance itself but of the lining (the epithelium) of the air tubes (bronchioles) in the lungs. Bronchial carcinoma – the medical term for lung cancer – starts in this epithelium. Researchers are, therefore, extremely interested in the epithelial cells that are present in coughed-up sputum. When cell division begins to go wrong – an early feature of a change in the direction of cancer – short lengths of DNA are left in the fluid within the epithelial cells. These fragments are called 'micronuclei' and the proportion of them is, of course, of great significance.

In a paper in the *British Journal of Cancer* at the end of 1992, the researcher Geert van Poppel and colleagues describe how the proportion of micronuclei in epithelial cells coughed up by smokers can be reduced by 30% by taking large doses of the antioxidant, beta-carotene.

This result, although of great scientific interest, has alarmed some of the scientists concerned with this problem. The epidemiologist, Professor Richard Peto, FRS, of the Imperial Cancer Research Fund in Oxford, is concerned that news about the value of antioxidants may lead smokers to believe that they can safely continue so long as they take their vitamins. He points out that it is still too early to say that DNA damage by free radicals is the most important reason for the high incidence of cancer in smokers. Whether it proves to be so or not, smoking will remain one of the most dangerous of human activities.

## *Stroke*

Stroke is the devastating consequence of a loss of the blood supply to a part of the brain so that damage occurs and the affected person is deprived, often permanently, of the full use of one or more of the brain functions – movement, sensation, speech, comprehension, vision, and so on. Threatened strokes are called transient ischaemic attacks (TIAs). These are mini-strokes lasting for less than 24 hours and then, apparently, reversing. Any of the manifestations of a full stroke may occur and TIAs are clear indications that one is at risk.

On 27 June 1992, the *Lancet* carried a paper from the Department of Neurology at Brussels University. This paper describes a study of 80 people who were showing definite signs of being at severe risk of developing a stroke. In this study, patients with TIAs lasting for more than three hours were matched against similar people who had never had TIAs, and the outcome assessed after 21 days. It was found that people with more than average vitamin A in their blood were significantly more likely to make a complete recovery than those with average amounts or less.

The trial also showed that those people whose symptoms and signs persisted for more than 24 hours, and whose blood levels of vitamin A were higher than average, ended up with less neurological damage than did those with low blood concentrations of the vitamin. Levels of vitamin E were assessed but no significant difference was found between those with below or above average concentrations of this vitamin.

Destruction of nerve cells in stroke and pre-stroke conditions is known to be partly due to oxidative damage by free radicals. The body does what it can to protect against these free radicals, but its capacity to do so is limited. Since you now know that vitamin E is highly effective in mopping up free radicals you may be wondering why it showed no useful effect in this case. Vitamin E works well in the presence of high concentrations of oxygen but not when there is a shortage of oxygen. Strokes and TIAs occur because not enough oxygen is reaching the nerve cells. Nerve cells in the brain have a higher rate of oxygen usage than any other cells in the body, and if there is any shortage as a result of reduced blood flow from narrowed arteries, available oxygen is quickly used up. Vitamin A, on the other hand, functions effectively as an antioxidant in conditions of low oxygen concentrations, and this may account for its apparent value in these cases. It is, of course, possible, that it also has valuable effects other than simply free radical trapping.

There is also the possibility that vitamin E will not pass through the walls of the smallest brain blood vessels – the capillaries – as easily as vitamin A. The brain capillaries are less permeable than those in other parts of the body. This is called the 'blood-brain barrier' and it prevents many substances, including some drugs, from getting through. Although vitamins A and E are both fat-soluble, the molecule of vitamin E is somewhat bulkier than that of vitamin A.

A lesson to be learned from this study would seem to be that each antioxidant has its optimum range of action, and that several different antioxidants are needed to ensure comprehensive cover. It would be foolish in the extreme, however, to suppose that taking antioxidant vitamins is an effective substitute for a healthy lifestyle that minimizes the risk factors for stroke – avoidance of smoking, good weight control, low intake of saturated fats, plenty of vegetables and fruit in the diet, and plenty of exercise.

## *Free radicals and Parkinson's disease*

Parkinson's disease, or *paralysis agitans*, is a progressively disabling condition featuring shaking of the hands with 'pill-rolling' finger movements, rigidity of muscles, slowness of speech and movements, difficulty in getting started in walking, tottering steps, a mask-like face and tiny handwriting. It is due to the degeneration of certain cells in the central part of the brain known as the 'substantia nigra' that produce a substance called 'dopamine'; and it is treated with the drug levodopa and other substances that stimulate dopamine receptors in the brain. The cause of the changes in the brain cells is unknown, but in the late 1980s it became clear that various oxidative processes involving the formation of free radicals were involved.

A large trial was therefore started in 1987 to see whether vitamin E in doses of 2,000 mg per day could delay the progress of the disease. Eight hundred patients with Parkinson's disease were involved in the trial, which was conducted simultaneously in a large number of different hospitals and research departments in America and Canada. The patients were divided into four groups, one of which received the vitamin E. The trial report was published in 1993 in the *New England Journal of Medicine*.

Unhappily, the trial showed no evidence of any beneficial effect of vitamin E on the progress of the disease. According to the researchers, this disappointing result might have been due to the fact that adequate amounts of the vitamin were unable to pass the 'blood-brain barrier' to reach the cells of the substantia nigra. It was also suggested that a negative result with vitamin E did not necessarily imply that other antioxidants might also be ineffective. They suggested that trials of these were still warranted. There were no significant adverse effects attributable to the dosage of the vitamin. One of the groups in the trial was treated with another drug, selegiline*(Eldepryl). This group did enjoy worthwhile benefit in terms of slowing of the disease.

Medical research can benefit from its failures as well as its successes. This major study teaches that theoretical ideas about free radicals are not always borne out in practice. The demonstration that free radicals are the cause of a particular kind of cell damage does not necessarily mean that any one particular antioxidant taken by mouth will prevent such damage. The antioxidant has to be appropriate and it has to get to the site of free radical damage.

## *Dupuytren's contracture of the hand*

Just to show that free radicals have been implicated in seemingly unlikely conditions, and that research into such conditions can throw light on the whole subject, I thought I would include this one. Dupuytren's contracture is a thickening and shortening of the fibrous layer below the skin of the palm of the hand, the palmar fascia, that leads to a fixed bending of the fingers into the palm, usually starting with the ring finger. It is surprisingly common, affecting between 4% and 6% of middle-aged men, rising to about 20% in men over 65.

In November 1987, Dr G. A. C. Murrell and colleagues of the Nuffield Department of Orthopaedic Surgery, Oxford University, published a paper in the *British Medical Journal* reporting the results of the measurement of free radical markers in samples of damaged palmar fascia removed at operation on patients with Dupuytren's contracture. The free radical markers were substances known as 'hypoxanthine' and 'xanthine', known to be implicated in the production of oxygen free radicals. Samples of normal fascia were obtained, to act as controls, from patients who did not have Dupuytren's contracture, but who were undergoing similar tissue removal operations for a different reason.

The samples taken from the Dupuytren's cases had six times the concentration of hypoxanthine as the control samples from people without Dupuytren's contracture. The researchers also confirmed the presence of the enzyme, xanthine oxidase, which

*available in India under the trade name deprenyl.

produces free radicals when acting on hypoxanthine. All this strongly suggested that free radicals were the cause of the contracture. The scientists went further, however, and in laboratory experiments on artificial cultures of the cells from the samples, showed that added free radicals in appropriate concentration caused the cells to increase greatly in number. These cells are called 'fibroblasts' and they produce the additional scar tissue that causes the contracture. Free radicals in excess killed the cells.

The drug, allopurinol, is known to be valuable in the management of Dupuytren's contracture. This drug acts by binding to the enzyme, xanthine oxidase, so that it cannot act on hypoxanthine to release free radicals.

## *Free radicals and AIDS*

It is interesting to note that people who are HIV-positive and are showing signs of AIDS have a much higher incidence of Dupuytren's contracture than HIV-negative people. In one series of articles, published in the *British Medical Journal* in 1990, 18 out of 50 HIV-positive men (36%) had established Dupuytren's contracture and another 6 were thought to have early thickening of the palm. One plausible reason for this extraordinarily high incidence of the condition in HIV-positive people may be that free radicals are produced in excessive amounts in such people. Increased amounts of the free radical marker, malonaldehyde has indeed been found in people with HIV infection. This was reported in the Scandinavian *Journal of Infectious Diseases* in 1988.

## *Phagocytes and free radicals*

The phagocytes (literally 'eating cells') are the scavengers of the body and do a wonderful job eating up and destroying undesirable substances and the germs that cause infection. They are mobile cells that are attracted to the site of infections or to foreign material by chemical stimuli. They are amoebic and get around by putting out long finger-like protrusions ('false feet' or pseudopodia) and flowing into them. This mobility also allows them to flow around anything they wish to destroy so that it is incorporated into their bodies. Inside the phagocytes are enzymes which, in the presence of bacteria and other organisms, produce the powerful oxygen free radical, superoxide. This immediately generates the strong oxidant, hydrogen peroxide. Hydrogen peroxide then acts on chloride in the phagocyte to form hypochlorous acid (the same stuff as Domestos), which soon copes with the germs.

Long-term inflammation means that successive waves of millions of phagocytes descend on the affected area of the body. Unfortunately, the free radicals do not stay in the phagocytes and large quantities are released into the surrounding tissues. Hydrogen peroxide and hypochlorous acid are profoundly damaging to body cells of all kinds and this is why inflammation is associated with tissue destruction. They also inflict damage on DNA and so can lead to cancer.

## *Red wine and free radicals*

For years, doctors have been embarrassed when asked why it is that the French, whose diet is high in saturated fats, nevertheless have a low incidence of the serious arterial disease, atherosclerosis (see p. 29) and a correspondingly low mortality from coronary heart disease. In medical circles, this is known as the 'French paradox'. Some medical people, especially those with a taste for wine, have maintained that this can somehow be attributed to a regular intake of red wine. The reasons they have given for this opinion have usually referred to the artery-widening (vasodilatation) effect of the alcohol content of the wine, and have not been found particularly plausible. A better suggestion has now been produced.

In the *British Medical Journal* for 20 February 1993, a paper appeared by scientists of the Lipid Research Group of the University of California. This paper referred to previous research that showed how oxidation of the cholesterol-carrying low-density lipoproteins (LDLs) allows cholesterol to be incorporated into the plaques of atherosclerosis in the walls of arteries (see p. 30). The paper then turned to a consideration of certain of the non-alcoholic constituents of the wine – several phenolic substances (flavonoids) which are known to have antioxidant properties.

Phenolics were prepared from Californian red wine and tested for their antioxidant powers on human low-density lipoproteins in the laboratory. These tests showed that the phenolic substances were even more effective than vitamin E in preventing the oxidation of LDLs. Wine diluted one thousand-fold, containing tiny quantities of phenolics, blocked the oxidation of LDLs significantly more than vitamin E. According to the authors, 'these data provide a plausible explanation for the French paradox'.

Since then, much research has shown that heart attacks and strokes are not the only medical benefits that wine can confer. It seems that the antioxidant effects of wine can have even wider effects. The *British Medical Journal* of 5 April 1997 reports French research that concluded that elderly people who drink wine in moderation were less likely to develop Alzheimer's disease or senile dementia than non-drinkers. In a nine-year study of 3,777 men and women over the age of 65 years, less than 1% of those who drank wine moderately developed dementia compared with 4.9% of non-drinkers and 5.1% of light drinkers. A moderate drinker in this series was defined as one who took three to four glasses a day. Another report, in the *Lancet* of 10 January 1998, describes research at Howard University, Washington DC, on the relationship between wine intake and the development of the distressing age-related condition of macular degeneration. This common disorder damages or destroys straight-ahead vision while leaving peripheral vision unaffected. The result may be that the sufferer is unable to read, recognize faces, tell the time, drive a car or enjoy television.

In a study of 3,072 adults over 45 years, a total of 184 were found to have macular degeneration. The remarkable thing was that 9% of those who did not drink developed the condition, while only 4% of those who drank wine regularly did so. After the figures were adjusted to eliminate the effects of a previous history of circulatory disease and other confusing factors, the wine-drinkers still came out with substantially less macular degeneration than the non-drinkers. This unexpected result was attributed to the antioxidant properties of wine and possibly, also, to its power of preventing blood platelets from sticking together and thus initiating a thrombosis.

The important point was made, however, that although a little of what you fancy can, apparently, do you good, more than moderate indulgence in wine will certainly bring its own problems, especially in older people.

## *Adult respiratory distress syndrome and free radicals*

The respiratory distress syndrome of adults is a serious and previously unpredictable complication of severe infection in which the lungs fill up with fluid and white cells and there is severe, often fatal, interference with the vital oxygenation of the blood. Recent research has shown that in this condition the balance of power between free radicals and natural body antioxidants changes in favour of the free radicals.

A report in the *Lancet* in March 1993 shows that measurement of certain of the body's natural antioxidants makes it possible to identify which people are most likely to develop this dangerous syndrome so that preventive treatment can be given. This study showed that 9 to 12 hours before the syndrome developed, the people concerned showed a definite rise in the amounts of superoxide dismutase and catalase (see p. 25) present in their bodies. This is a clear indication of increased free radical activity giving warning of impending trouble. Since free radicals are now implicated in so many different conditions, it seems likely that anticipatory investigations of this kind may become more important in the future.

## *The expansion of medical interest in free radicals*

The March 1993 paper in the *Lancet* is just another example of the reports of free radical research now appearing regularly in the professional medical press. Other conditions in which free radicals have been implicated or suspected of being important include:

- pressure sores;
- red blood cell damage;
- paraquat poisoning;

- carbon tetrachloride poisoning;
- ozone damage;
- skeletal muscle damage;
- liver cell damage;
- spinal cord injury;
- diabetes;
- possibly cancer caused by electromagnetic fields from power lines.

Free radicals have also been found to be active in alcohol toxicity and in bringing about the tumour-destructive action of anticancer drugs.

Papers on free radicals have appeared in numerous medical and other journals from all over the world. Here are a few, in addition to those already mentioned, that have published articles on the subject: *Acta Physiologica Scandinavica, American Journal of Clinical Nutrition, American Journal of Epidemiology, Annals of Clinical Biochemistry, Annals of the Royal College of Surgeons of England, Biochemical Medicine, Cancer Research, Free Radical Biology and Medicine, Gastroenterology, International Journal of Epidemiology, Journal of the American College of Cardiology, Journal of Biological Chemistry, Journal of Inorganic Biochemistry, Journal of Pharmacology, Nature* and *Toxicology and Applied Pharmacology.*

With this much serious medical and scientific interest in the subject, can you really afford to ignore it?

# 8
# All About Antioxidant Vitamins

Most current medical textbooks still treat vitamins, including vitamin C and vitamin E, in the conventional manner. This is appropriate for the large B group of vitamins ($B_1$, $B_2$, $B_6$ and $B_{12}$, niacin, pantothenic acid, folic acid and lipoic acid) and for vitamins A, D and K. All these, plus vitamin C, are substances necessary in very small quantities for the maintenance of health. If these small quantities are not available, various deficiency diseases occur. Vitamin C deficiency causes scurvy – a bleeding disorder; vitamin A deficiency causes serious eye and other problems; vitamin D deficiency causes bone softening – rickets or osteomalacia; and so on.

## *Danger of overdosage*

Because many vitamins act in association with enzymes and only tiny quantities are required, it has become conventional to teach that people who take more than the small daily requirement – which is nearly always present in a reasonably balanced diet – are wasting their money. In addition, there have been regular, and well-justified, medical warnings about the dangers of vitamin overdosage, specifically of vitamins A and D. Excessive intake of these vitamins can certainly cause trouble. The dangers of vitamin A overdosage are described below, as are those of Vitamin E.

Although few textbooks have yet got around to the role of certain vitamins as biological antioxidants, there is plenty about this in the current medical and general scientific literature. Textbooks take a long time to write, edit and publish and they invariably lag behind current advances, especially in new and rapidly developing fields of research. This is why medical and scientific journals are so important. In the free radicals literature most of the emphasis has been on vitamins E and C, so it is worth looking more closely at these interesting substances.

## *Vitamin E (tocopherol)*

Until recently, pharmacology textbooks have dismissed the fat-soluble vitamin E as unimportant; some have even said that it is of no medical relevance in humans. Tocopherol was first discovered in 1922 when it was found that female rats required an unknown substance in their diets to sustain normal pregnancies. Without it, they could ovulate and conceive satisfactorily, but within about 10 days the fetuses invariably died and were absorbed. Male rats deficient in this substance were also found to have abnormalities in their testes. For these reasons, vitamin E enjoyed a brief reputation as the 'anti-sterility vitamin' and was, illogically, recommended as a treatment for infertility, although there was no reason to suppose that the people concerned were deficient in the vitamin. This was the kind of thinking that gave megavitamin therapy a bad name with the medical profession.

Vitamin E has also been used to try to treat various menstrual disorders, inflammation of the vagina and menopausal symptoms, but there is no evidence that it is of any value in these conditions.

Vitamin E was first isolated in 1936 from wheatgerm oil. It was found to be any one of a range of eight very complicated but similar molecules known as 'tocopherols'. It is almost insoluble in water but dissolves in oils, fats, alcohol, acetone, ether and other fat solvents. Unlike vitamin C. it is stable to heat and alkalis in the absence of oxygen and is unaffected by acids at temperatures up to 100°C. If exposed to atmospheric oxygen, it is slowly oxidized. This occurs more rapidly in the presence of iron or silver salts. It gradually darkens on exposure to light. Among the richest natural sources are seed germ oils, alfalfa and lettuce. It is widely distributed in plant materials. The international unit is equal to 1 mg of alpha-tocopherol acetate. Because there are eight tocopherols, natural vitamin E varies a little in its strength. But for practical purposes of dosage you can consider 1 international unit to be equivalent to 1 mg.

All the tocopherols are antioxidants, and this appears to be the basis for all the biological effects of the vitamin. It is now becoming increasingly clear that vitamin E is involved in many body processes and that it operates as a natural antioxidant helping to protect important cell structures, especially the cell membranes, from the damaging effects of free radicals. Interestingly, it has been found, for instance, that the vitamin can protect against the effects of overdosage of vitamin A. In animals, vitamin E supplements can protect them against the effects of various drugs, chemicals and metals that can promote free radical formation. In carrying out its function as an antioxidant in the body, vitamin E is, itself, converted to a radical. It is, however, soon regenerated to the active vitamin by a biochemical process that probably involves both vitamin C and glutathione.

Real deficiency of vitamin E is very rare because it occurs widely in food, especially in vegetable oils, but when it does occur the effects can be devastating. The need for vitamin E increases if the diet is high in polyunsaturated fats. Deficiency sometimes occurs in premature babies, especially if malnourished, and in people with disorders that interfere with fat absorption. People who are severely deficient in vitamin E for these reasons may suffer, to varying degrees, from:

- degenerative changes in the brain and nervous system;
- impairment of vision;
- double vision;
- walking disturbances;
- anaemia;
- an increased rate of destruction of red blood cells;
- fluid retention (oedema);
- skin disorders.

Some reports have shown that large doses of vitamin E can prevent the progression of the neurological abnormalities or even lead to improvement.

Human vitamin E deficiency occurs only after many months on a severely deficient diet. A daily intake of 10 to 30 mg of the vitamin is said to be sufficient to keep the blood levels within 'normal' limits and this will always be provided by a normal diet. Diets that contain other antioxidants decrease the requirement. Human milk contains plenty to meet the baby's needs.

## *Dangers of overdosage*

Vitamin E is generally regarded as being a fairly innocuous substance and few if any warnings are heard of the dangers of overdosage. For adults, this is probably reasonable, but there are undoubtedly limits to the amounts that can be safely taken. Cases have occurred in which dangers have arisen from overdosage of vitamin E in premature babies from probable interference with the action of cells of the immune system against infection.

Since free radical oxidant action is a necessary part of the body's functioning, both for the destruction of bacteria and for other important purposes, it is only reasonable to suppose that undue interference with it, by excessive dosage of an antioxidant like vitamin E, is likely to be harmful. To do so may be, for instance, to increase the risk of infection. There is no substance of major medical benefit that does not also carry the risk of undesirable side effects. This is a fact of medical life that should never be forgotten.

Like many other substances, vitamin E is necessary for life and health. But, like many other substances, the amount in the body must, for safety, be kept within fairly strict limits.

## *Vitamin C (ascorbic acid)*

Vitamin C is a simpler compound than vitamin E and is water-soluble. It was the first vitamin to be discovered, and the disease caused by its deficiency – scurvy – has been known for centuries. Sailors on long sea voyages, who subsisted on salt pork and biscuits with no fresh fruit or vegetables, used commonly to die of scurvy. They became listless, debilitated, and anaemic. Their legs swelled up and their gums bled and became spongy and ulcerated. Their teeth fell out, there was bleeding into their skins and mucous membranes, and their condition quickly worsened and they died.

But in 1747, the British naval doctor, James Lind (1716–84) proved by careful experiments, with controls, that a teaspoonful of lemon juice, taken from time to time, would prevent the disease. Unfortunately, it was 50 years before their lordships of the Admiralty – who were not readily impressed by science –

could be persuaded to issue appropriate orders to their ships' captains, and in the meantime many more sailors died.

The vitamin was isolated in 1928 and chemically identified in 1932. It is readily destroyed by exposure to air and by cooking, especially in the presence of copper and alkalis. The main structural material of the body is a protein called 'collagen'. This forms the main basis of the bones and of most other tissues. Vitamin C is necessary for the proper synthesis of collagen, and deficiency leads to the failure of wounds to heal, and weakness and rupture of small blood vessels and of all the collagen tissues of the body. Scurvy still occurs in people who live on a diet exclusively of tea and buns. The first symptoms appear three or four months after the last intake of the vitamin. In babies and small children, scurvy also causes bleeding under the bone membranes giving rise to very tender swellings so that the affected infants resent being touched.

To prevent scurvy, humans need amounts of the vitamin varying from about 60 mg a day to as much as 250 mg a day. People who smoke and those on the contraceptive pill need more than others. People need more while suffering from infectious diseases, injuries, burns, rheumatic disorders and after surgical operations. A normal, well-balanced diet will usually supply enough vitamin C to prevent scurvy. The vitamin is plentiful in fruit juices, green peppers, cabbages, greens, potatoes, citrus fruits, tomatoes and strawberries. Orange and lemon juices contain about 0.5 mg in each cc (ml). When large doses are taken, there is a correspondingly large loss of the vitamin in the urine.

Vitamin C is a powerful antioxidant and is commonly used for this reason to preserve the natural flavour and colour of processed fruit, fruit drinks, vegetables and dairy products.

## *The value of vitamin C in medicine*

No one disputes that vitamin C is of great value in the treatment of scurvy. As soon as the vitamin is given in adequate dosage, improvement occurs and, within a few weeks, all the symptoms and signs have gone. The real dispute has been whether the vitamin has any value in people who are not suffering from scurvy. Until about ten tears ago, the orthodox medical view was that if you get enough to prevent scurvy, additional intake of the vitamin is a waste of time and money and does no good.

Oddly enough, in spite of this view, there have been, over the years, repeated enthusiasms for trials of the vitamin in all sorts of conditions. Even before the current interest in free radicals and in the use of antioxidants, vitamin C had many respectable supporters. One reason for the medical scepticism is clear; most of the trials of vitamin C in the management of conditions like the common cold failed because the doses given were very little more than the minimum daily requirement to prevent scurvy. It is becoming clear that, used as an antioxidant, much larger doses than the minimum daily requirement are needed.

## *Possible dangers*

Vitamin C has an excellent safety record and has been taken in 1,000 mg (1 gram) plus doses by millions of people with no apparent disadvantage. To balance this there has been a handful of reports of ill effects of very large doses thought to be due to the vitamin.

One of these was published in the *British Medical Journal* in March 1993. This paper reports the case of a 32-year-old HIV-positive man who developed generalized lymph node enlargement. He was advised by his doctors to start AZT treatment but refused and sought the advice of a medically qualified nutritionist. Investigation showed that he had a lower than normal blood level of the antioxidant, glutathione, and he was prescribed, among other things, glutathione supplements and a course of vitamin C to be given in a dosage of 40,000 mg (40 grams) by intravenous injection, three times a week, plus 20,000 to 40,000 mg (20 to 40 grams) every day by mouth. This enormous dosage was continued for a month with no obvious change in his condition. The intravenous dose was then doubled to 80,000 mg (80 grams). The next day he became breathless and feverish and his urine turned to a black colour, indicating that many red blood cells had broken down, releasing haemoglobin which was passing out in the urine, much in the manner of malarial 'blackwater fever'.

Investigation showed that this man had sickle-cell trait and a comparatively rare genetic blood disorder known as 'glucose-6-phosphate dehydrogenase deficiency'. This enzyme deficiency disorder makes red blood cells much more fragile than normal because of a shortage of the antioxidant, glutathione, which protects the red cells against free radical damage. Many drugs in common use can cause the red cells to break down in this condition. The patient was given lots of fluid to drink so as to flush through his kidneys, and on the third day the urine was clear. He made a complete recovery from the red blood cell breakdown.

Dosages of this order are ridiculously high and there are very few remedies that can, with perfect safety, be taken in quantities of 20 or 30 times the customary dosage. This patient was receiving dosages of about 500 times the recommended daily allowance. The report does, however, indicate that there are some people who ought to be particularly cautious about taking any drug, even one as apparently safe as vitamin C.

In April 1998 a research report appeared in the journal *Nature*. This was an account of a study at the University of Leicester by a team headed by Dr Ian Podmore. DNA contains four bases – guanine, adenine, thymine and cytosine – and it is the order of these along the DNA chain that is the genetic code. Dr Podmore's research measured the amounts of guanine and adenine that had been damaged by oxidation. Thirty healthy volunteers were given 500 mg of vitamin C every day and the levels of oxidized guanine and adenine were measured. As might be expected, the levels of oxidized guanine did fall.

The important point, however, is that those of oxidized adenine actually rose. After stopping the vitamin dosage the levels of both of these markers of oxidation fell back to normal within seven weeks. DNA is being attacked all the time by free radicals and is constantly being repaired. Evidence that vitamin C can apparently increase oxidative damage to one of the four bases of DNA is puzzling. Should we conclude from this that vitamin C can be harmful? At this stage we cannot answer this question. The best we can do is to try to balance this finding against the mass of epidemiological and other evidence supporting the beneficial effects of vitamin C. Then we must make up our own minds.

## *Beta-carotene*

The antioxidant plant pigment beta-carotene is also known as 'provitamin A' because it is converted into vitamin A (retinol and other forms) in the liver. It is found in whole milk, butter, cheese, egg yolk, liver, yellow and green vegetables and fish, especially in the liver. The same foods also contain a number of different carotene-like substances (carotenoids) that cannot be converted to vitamin A and so are wasted.

Retinol and its related substances have many important functions in the body. They are necessary for:

- growth and health of the surface and lining tissues and the bones;
- health of the immune system;
- protection against cancer;
- normal vision;
- health of the corneas;
- protection against various skin diseases;
- protection of the skin against sunlight radiation;
- protection against ageing changes.

People deficient in retinoids suffer night blindness and dryness of the eyes (xerophthalmia). In the case of babies, they may suffer devastating melting of the corneas of the eyes with permanent blindness. Severe deficiency is a common cause of death in small children after severe damage has been sustained by most systems of the body.

A normal, well-balanced diet will provide quite enough retinol to prevent any such effects. If taken as a dietary supplement, 1 mg per day is equivalent to the recommended daily allowance and this dose is probably double the amount needed to prevent deficiency.

Remember that vitamin A or its provitamin, beta-carotene, is not in the same safe category as vitamins C and E. No one who knows anything about the matter would ever think of recommending megadoses of vitamin A.

# 9
# Your Challenge

If you have read carefully to this point, you are now in possession of all the important current knowledge on free radicals and antioxidant vitamins. Of course, there are many additional things in the scientific literature that I might have included. But if I had done that you might have found the book confusing or hard to read, so I thought it better to select.

In writing a book of this kind it is difficult to avoid personal bias. Over the years I have formed some firm opinions on the matter and it is important for me to concentrate on putting across facts rather than opinions. Nothing is easier than to deliberately select those reports and arguments that support a particular point of view and to ignore or play down those that do not. To do this is neither honest nor safe. At the same time, it is impossible to research and study a subject as potentially important as this without taking up a position. Once this has happened it becomes even more difficult to be disinterested. So I have had to be careful not to give way to a natural tendency to accentuate the evidence in favour and I am not sure that I have entirely succeeded.

You will have gathered that I have long been convinced of the importance of free radicals and of the value of antioxidant vitamin treatment. Whatever they may say about Linus Pauling, I am on his side. It is a matter of great regret to me that he died (at a very advanced age) before I could send him a copy of a book of this kind. I would have liked to have been able to think of him with his large jar of vitamin C on his desk, munching away while reading this book, hopefully with approval.

I am reasonably sure that I have not made any claims that are not well supported by scientific evidence. One must, of course, take on trust the statements made in the various reports and made verbally by scientific enthusiasts. This is not so hazardous as you might think. Published scientific work is closely and critically scrutinized by many other scientists, especially those working in the same field, and the one thing they are looking for are claims or assertions that they think may not be backed up by convincing evidence. All really important findings are independently checked by repeated research, done by other people, and many papers are published to refute or confirm such work.

## *Be sceptical*

Having declared my interest, I am now going to summarize the arguments and challenge you to make up your own mind on the matter. I hope you will read what follows with scepticism. In particular, you should be wary of believing that just because something follows something else, the second must necessarily be a consequence of the first. Let me give you an example of what I mean.

I used to suffer wretchedly from repeated colds, often every two or three weeks. Years ago, I started to take 1,000 mg of vitamin C every day and, whenever a cold seemed to be threatening, I increased the dosage to 2,000 or 3,000 mg daily. Since then I have hardly ever had an established cold and, almost always, find that I can abort a threatened cold with the extra dosage.

This is not proof. On this basis alone, I am not entitled to believe that it is the vitamin C that is preventing the colds. Other things may have happened, coincidentally with my starting to take the vitamin, that increased my resistance to colds. When I became a full-time writer I changed my lifestyle and came in contact with far fewer people. This could have been the cause. It is even possible that my expectation of benefit from vitamin C brings this about by some obscure psychological effect on my immune system.

But if, at the same time, I have evidence that the viruses that cause colds do their cellular damage by producing free radicals (I don't actually know this, but it could be true), and that vitamin C can mop up free radicals, then I am entitled to have more confidence in the idea that vitamin C prevents colds. Since I have no evidence that viruses produce free radicals, I must continue to consider the matter 'not proven'. The Romans recognized the logical fallacy of believing that because one event follows another the former must have been the cause of the latter. They called it the *post hoc ergo propter hoc* fallacy ('after this, therefore because of this'). This is one of the commonest forms of logical error, and we are all prone to it.

The many important facts presented to you in this book have been scattered between the chapters. It seems useful, therefore, to bring them all together in a brief summary, expressed in a slightly different way, so that you can pick up any points you have missed.

## *The argument*

Cells are the tiny, microscopic units of which the body is made. Cells are living, highly active units, busily engaged in carrying out thousands of chemical reactions concerned with energy production, protein synthesis, growth and repair, material storage, information transmission, hormone production, making poisons and drugs safe, and so on. Similar cells stick join together to form simple tissues, these form more complex tissues, tissues form organs, and organs form systems.

Disease is any impairment of the structure or the function of cells. So it can affect single cells, tissues, organs, whole systems or the whole body. Until comparatively recently, the actual way in which the molecules of body cells are injured in disease was unknown. We knew a great deal about the changes that occur in cells in the course of disease but little about the way in which this was brought about. We also knew how important the outer layer of the cell – the cell membrane – was, and how often disease processes resulted in damage to this membrane. The cell membrane is made mainly of fatty tissue, including cholesterol. We also knew that disease processes damage other parts of the cell, including the tiny cell organs (organelles) such as the mitochondria that produce energy, and the DNA at the centre of the cell (the nucleus).

We now know that a very important way in which cell membranes and other parts of the cell can be damaged is by the chemical reactions that occur between the molecules of the cell and a class of short-lived but highly active chemical groups known as 'oxygen free radicals'. This chemical reaction is known as 'oxidation' – a kind of burning – and it is always damaging to the substances oxidized. Free radicals also convert normal body molecules into free radicals and thus often start chain reactions which multiply the damage.

At about the same time as this was discovered, it was also found that the body has its own, built-in systems for combatting free radicals. These are normal body constituents, known as 'antioxidants', and their job is to get rid of excess free radicals. They do this by altering them slightly so that they cease to be chemically active and become harmless. More than half a dozen of these natural antioxidants are known. One of them is vitamin E, usually called 'alpha-tocopherol' (see p. 81). It is very rare for anyone to be severely deficient in vitamin E, but when this happens, almost every part of the body suffers serious damage. The killing and scavenging cells of our immune system (phagocytes) use free radicals to destroy the germs they have absorbed. At least in very small babies, too much vitamin E can interfere with this action and allow infection to get the upper hand. So we know that in some cases it is possible to have too much vitamin E.

Vitamin E does not dissolve in water but does dissolve in fat. Cell membranes and low-density lipoproteins are largely made of the fatty material, cholesterol. Vitamin E is probably the only antioxidant that can fix itself to cell membranes and to LDLs. So it seems probable that this is the main protective substance against cell membrane and LDL oxidation damage.

The body also reacts badly to a deficiency of vitamin C (scurvy) but the effects of this are much less widespread than those of a deficiency of vitamin E. Vitamin C, however, is a powerful antioxidant and is soluble in water, so it makes its way to every part of the body – which is over 90% water. All the cells of the body contain water and all are bathed in water. The amount of vitamin C in the body varies considerably with the diet and doses up to about 10,000 mg (10 grams) a day are almost certainly harmless.

Many hundreds of medical and scientific papers have now been published showing that various disease conditions are associated with free radicals. Hundreds have also been published showing that if the body is low in antioxidants, especially vitamin E, vitamin C and beta-carotene, the affected person is more likely to suffer from various diseases other than the known vitamin-deficiency diseases. So far, the strongest evidence is in connection with the serious artery disease, atherosclerosis, which causes heart attacks, strokes and gangrene and is the largest single cause of death in the Western world. Free radicals have actually been detected (a very difficult thing to do) following heart attacks. There is also convincing evidence that low antioxidant levels promote the eye disease, cataract. Good evidence also exists that free radicals are strongly implicated in the cellular changes occurring in ageing, in the damage caused by smoking and in the destructive effects of sunlight on the skin. We know that free radicals can damage DNA and there are grounds, less secure than for other conditions, for the belief that they are implicated in the development of at least some cancers. Low antioxidant levels in men are associated with increased birth defects in their children.

Cigarette smoking causes a substantial drop in the levels of antioxidants in the bodies of smokers. This is believed to be because cigarette smoke contains so many free radicals and promotes so many additional free radicals in the body that much of the antioxidant potential is used up coping with these. As a result, cigarette smokers are more heavily under attack from free radicals than non-smokers. There is a wealth of evidence for the view that the wide spectrum of increased disease and premature mortality suffered by smokers is largely due to the action of free radicals.

## *The challenge*

You will have noticed that I have not referred here to the obvious next stage – trials to see whether heart disease, stroke, cancer, cataract, and so on can actually be prevented by taking antioxidant vitamins. There is a good reason for this. It is impossible to tell for certain whether someone is going to be spared such diseases until they are actually dead. Such trials, therefore, must inevitably take many years. Many major trials have, however, already been done and many more are in progress. To date, results have supported the view that the antioxidant vitamins C and E can do you a power of good. There is really no evidence that they can do you any harm.

This is where the challenge comes in. Unless you are very young, there is not much point is waiting ten years or so for proof that you should have been doing something really important for the last ten years. You really have to make up your mind now, and I am challenging you to do so.

If all these clever and dedicated scientific researchers – many from the world's most prestigious research institutions and universities – are wrong, and this free radical business is all nonsense, then you do have quite a lot to lose. Between 1,000 and 2,000 mg of vitamin C and 200 to 400 mg of vitamin E a day are going to cost you less than Rs 100 per month – maybe less if you shop around. Vitamin C is very cheap, but unless done up in waxy, coated tablets or in a flavoured, fizzy formulation, is horribly sour and you will soon get discouraged. These fancy preparations are, unfortunately, more expensive than the basic acid.

I don't think you need worry about any harmful side effects of such dosage as I have just mentioned, as millions of people have already proved. It is possible that the very occasional sensitive person might show what is called an 'idiosyncratic reaction' of some kind. Such things do happen. If you do notice any such harmful effect, stop the tablets and capsules. You will also have to watch your intake of vitamin A – not by taking lots of pills, which could be dangerous, but by ensuring that your diet is adequate.

But suppose these scientists are right and all the evidence they have produced means what they think it means. In that case, it is true that free radicals are, at this very moment, attacking and oxidizing your low-density lipoproteins so that they are damaging the walls of your arteries, clogging them up with atheromatous plaques and cutting down the vital blood supply to your heart, brain, other organs and limbs. It is true that whenever you are exposed to sunlight, the collagen in your skin is being attacked and degraded by radiation-induced free radicals so that it can no longer maintain youthful smoothness and elasticity or provide the support that prevents wrinkling and broken veins.

It is true that, as you read, the protein in the internal lenses of your eyes is being oxidized and changed so that cataracts may form. Perhaps worst of all, it is true that the DNA in many of the cells of your body is being attacked and damaged by free radicals so that the race is on between the rate of damage and the processes of repair. If the free radicals win, the result may simply be the death of some cells, which is of no great consequence. But it may also be a DNA mutation that could proceed to a cancerous change in a cell or, in the case of the sperm-producing cells, a genetic mutation that could be passed on to the children.

So it is up to you.

One last and very important point. If you are convinced that this kind of self-treatment actually does work, you might be tempted to use it as a substitute for healthy living, and especially as a justification for continuing to smoke. You could hardly make a more serious mistake. Antioxidant treatment may well turn out to be of major health importance, but it can never be a substitute for healthy living.

# 10

# Questions and Answers About Antioxidants and Free Radicals

**Q. How much vitamin C should I take?**

**A.** I don't know. I don't think anyone knows, for sure. What I do know, however, is that although the present official recommended minimum daily allowance is probably enough to stop you from getting scurvy (see p. 84), it isn't going to be much good for anything else. In certain circumstances it might not even prevent deficiency problems. The trouble is that the body's antioxidant needs are constantly changing. If your cells are especially under attack because of an infection or because you are on certain drugs or have inhaled a lot of car exhaust fumes or because you are a smoker, or even because you have accidentally taken some poisonous substance, then you will need a lot more than the basic amount – whatever that is. The big trials under way should show what sort of dosage can cover most eventualities. I suspect that 1,000 mg a day should be considered a basic dose and that you should increase this temporarily to 2,000 mg or 3,000 mg if you think you are at special risk.

**Q. What do you mean, 'at risk'?**

**A.** If you get a slight sore throat or any other indication of a cold, increase the daily dose. Similarly, if you feel unwell and suspect that you are 'sickening' for anything. Things like that. I suppose the time will come when we will up the intake for any early sign of indisposition or minor injury of any kind. Don't imagine, however, that an extra dose of vitamin C is any substitute for proper medical attention when this is obviously needed. Solid vitamin C tablets are also probably not a very good idea if you suffer from peptic ulcers or severe dyspepsia. In such cases, use a soluble preparation.

**Q. What is the best preparation of vitamin C?**

**A.** I recommend that you go for tablets which can be chewed or swallowed easily. Chewable tablets are also available in different flavours which camouflage the sour taste of vitamin C. It is almost impossible to eat plain ascorbic acid powder.

**Q. Some vitamin C tablets also contain flavonoids. Is this good?**

**A.** Flavonoids are also antioxidant, but the presence of flavonoids might, theoretically, limit the safe dose of the vitamin C tablet. Unless you are taking very large doses, the presence of flavonoids shouldn't matter.

**Q. Is it true that some animals make their own vitamin C?**

**A.** Yes. In fact, only humans, other apes, primates, guinea pigs and some bats are unable to synthesize vitamin C. Animals make it from glucose, but we lack the liver enzyme to carry out the last stage in the process. This suggests that earlier in evolution we were able to make the vitamin but that a mutation occurred in the common ancestor of the primates, maybe around 25 million years ago, so that the gene for this enzyme was deleted.

**Q. I understand the body stores vitamin C. Is this true?**

**A.** Yes. Most people who are not taking supplementary vitamin C have a store of about 1,500 mg or more. If you take an additional daily dose, the store will reach about 2,500 mg and you will start to pass more vitamin C in the urine.

**Q. Does a lot of vitamin C pass out in the urine?**

**A.** Yes. Vitamin C is rapidly lost from the body into the urine. In people saturated with vitamin C, the average half-life of the vitamin, after a 1 gram dose, is 3.37 hours. That means that after 3.37 hours after absorbing 1,000 mg, only an additional 500 mg will be left in the body. In 7 hours only about an additional 250 mg will be left and in 11 hours, only about an additional 125 mg will remain. Saturation means the presence in the body of a total of about 2.5 grams (2,500 mg) of vitamin C. Amounts above this level will be excreted as described. You don't need to take a lot of vitamin C to maintain saturation. Less than 250 mg per day will do it. The clinical evidence, however, implies that the best antioxidant effect requires levels above saturation.

**Q. Doesn't this suggest that sustained-release tablets of vitamin C are better? Is there any advantage in those?**

**A.** Sustained-release tablets may even out the levels above saturation, but we don't know whether this is beneficial. You will probably do just as well to take ordinary tablets twice or thrice a day.

**Q. But don't these large fluctuations in body levels affect the efficiency of the antioxidant effect?**

**A.** This is possible. But we don't really know. Many of the people in the successful trials are on once-a-day dosage. If you have reason to believe that free radicals are attacking, that is the time to take a supplementary dose so as to hit them hard.

**Q. What happens to the body levels when single doses much larger than 1 gram are taken by mouth?**

**A.** A good question. After taking a single dose of 1 gram, 75% of the dose is absorbed. The proportion absorbed decreases steadily with increasing dosage, until, with a 5 gram dose, only 20% (one-fifth) is absorbed. This sounds like being on a hiding to nothing. But remember that the statement refers to a single oral dose, not to the total daily dose. It also reinforces the advantages of multiple doses over single daily doses.

**Q. I have been offered, at a low price, a large stock of rather old vitamin C tablets that are turning brown. Should I buy them?**

**A.** No. Vitamin C is an unstable compound that darkens on exposure to light. Being an antioxidant it is not at all happy in an atmosphere of oxygen and deteriorates rapidly in air. It should be stored in airtight containers, preferably glass and protected from light. It is also readily destroyed by heat and alkalis.

**Q. What about allergy to vitamin C? Does this occur?**

**A.** This is very rare but has been reported in a few patients with strong allergic tendencies (atopy). It may present as asthma, eczema or as nettle rash (urticaria). Atopic people are advised to take any new preparation in a small dose initially and to look out for allergic effects over a period before starting on full dosage.

**Q. Is vitamin C excreted in breast milk?**

**A.** Yes. This soluble substance is rapidly distributed throughout the body. Human breast milk contains from 30 to 55 mg of vitamin C per litre. This means that, on average, a breastfed baby gets about 35 mg a day of vitamin C. This is the recommended minimum daily allowance.

**Q. Does it get through the placenta to the fetus in pregnant women?**

**A.** Yes.

**Q. So does it harm the fetus?**

**A.** The only reported adverse effect is of what is called 'rebound scurvy' in babies born to mothers taking high doses of the vitamin. There was a single report about this in an American pharmacology journal in 1977, but not much, if anything, seems to have been published on this effect since then. Bearing in mind the millions of people taking vitamin C supplements (said to be about 8% of the entire US population) and the extreme rarity of such reports, this must be very uncommon. Nevertheless, it is always necessary to exercise great care in taking any form of medication during pregnancy. Doses larger than those recommended should be avoided in pregnancy.

**Q. Is vitamin C used as an antioxidant other than in the body?**

**A.** Yes. Its antioxidant properties are extensively used to preserve the flavour, colour and general acceptability of a wide range of foods, especially dairy products and processed fruit and vegetables.

**Q. Vitamin E doses are given in IU not mg. What are IU?**

**A.** International units. Vitamin E, in practice, is not a pure substance but a mixture of tocopherols, of which there are eight or so. You will not go far wrong if you count international units as mg (milligrams). 1 mg of alpha-tocopherol acetate – the commonest form – is equal to one international unit.

**Q. What are carotenoids?**

**A.** These are the substances found in plants, fish liver, other liver, dairy products, etc. that are converted by the human liver into vitamin A. Beta-carotene is the most active carotenoid found in plants. There is growing evidence that, quite apart from their rolc as provitamin A, carotenoids can prevent, or help to prevent, various diseases.

**Q. Can they prevent cancer?**

**A.** I don't know for sure. There is plenty of statistical evidence that if you take a large group of people all with high levels of beta-carotene in their blood, and compare them with an equal group with low levels of beta-carotene, the first group will have fewer cases of cancer than the second, especially lung cancer. This has been reported in the *British Journal of Cancer* and in the medical journal *Cancer*. This doesn't prove that beta-carotene prevents cancer. It seems likely, however, that it makes you less likely to get some kinds of cancer.

**Q. Is this an antioxidant effect?**

**A.** Very likely. Beta-carotene is a powerful antioxidant that mops up free radicals produced by radiation or by various cancer-producing substances (carcinogens). These free radicals can cause DNA mutations that can lead to cancer. Moreover, a shortage of beta-carotene has, for some time, been known to lead to particular changes in surface cells (epithelia) characteristic of early cancer. The administration of beta-carotene reverses these early changes.

**Q. Is vitamin A fat-soluble?**

**A.** Yes. Vitamins A, D, E and K are fat-soluble; C is water-soluble.

**Q. Does the solubility matter?**

**A.** Yes. Fat-soluble antioxidants stay in cell membranes, which are made of two layers of fat molecules, and in low-density lipoproteins (see p. 32 ). Water-soluble vitamins may be present in the water in the cell or in the water surrounding the cell, but not in the membrane. Remember that antioxidants must get very close to the point of free radical production if they are to work.

**Q. What happens when free radicals attack a cell membrane?**

**A.** Hydroxyl free radicals have a voracious appetite for electrons and immediately hunt out unsaturated (double) bonds in the fatty acids of the membrane fats. When one of these bonds is broken, the molecule is split and the parts will have unpaired electrons (see p. 19 ). That means that they are now, themselves, free radicals. These, in turn, attack other fatty acid bonds, so a chain reaction can zip through the cell membrane causing terrible damage and even killing the cell.

**Q. So which free radicals does vitamin E deal with – the original cause of the chain reaction or those in the membrane?**

**A.** Vitamin E is a brilliant scavenger of split-fat-molecule free radicals, and if present, does a great job in stopping chain reactions and saving cells.

**Q. If a vitamin E molecule picks up an unpaired electron, doesn't this convert vitamin E into a free radical?**

**A.** Quite right. It does. Fortunately, the normal vitamin E molecule is quickly regenerated.

**Q. How?**

**A.** The biochemistry is complicated and, so far as I know, is not fully worked out.

But it seems to involve vitamin C and the natural antioxidant, glutathione. Incidentally, the enzyme glutathione peroxidase (see p. 25) is also important in removing peroxidized fatty acids from cell membranes.

**Q. Does this mean that if we are taking vitamin E, we should also take vitamin C?**

**A.** Yes. But I believe we should be taking vitamin C, anyhow, for all sorts of other reasons.

**Q. Are people who don't eat leafy green and yellow vegetables more liable to suffer certain diseases, such as cancer, than people who do?**

**A.** The evidence of a considerable number of surveys certainly suggests so.

**Q. Is this because of the protective effect of antioxidant vitamins?**

**A.** That is the general presumption. Judging by the medical literature, this presumption is shared by most of the experts.

**Q. How does vitamin E work?**

**A.** Vitamin E, being fat-soluble, settles in cell membranes and in low-density lipoproteins (see p. 32). Its molecule carries a hydroxyl group (see p. 20) from which the hydrogen atom is easily removed. This contributes the single electron needed to fill the outer orbital of any nearby free radical and render it harmless. This, of course, turns the vitamin E molecule into a free radical, but apparently it can move to the surface of the cell membrane or LDL globule where it reacts with vitamin C and is restored to normal.

**Q. What happens when molecules are oxidized?**

**A.** First, two oxygen atoms, linked together to form an oxygen molecule, approach the target molecule. Then an electron is transferred from the target molecule onto the oxygen molecule. This turns the oxygen molecule into a superoxide free radical, avid to link on to something. And, of course, the thing it latches on to is the target molecule, changing it to a quite different compound – an oxide.

**Q. In what way different?**

**A.** As different as rust is from iron or quicklime is from chalk, or laughing gas is from nitrogen. Oxides have quite different properties from the parent substance before it was oxidized.

**Q. But oxidation is essential to life. Does this mean that superoxide free radicals are essential to life?**

**A.** Yes. But the enzyme that makes them safe – superoxide dismutase (see p. 25) is also essential to life. Bacteria have been genetically engineered so that the gene for superoxide dismutase was removed. They all died.

**Q. Has there ever been a case reported of a deficiency of superoxide dismutase in humans?**

**A.** Not that I know of. This would almost certainly be a lethal mutation causing death at a very early stage after conception.

**Q. Is it actually possible to detect free radicals?**

**A.** Yes, but it's not easy.

**Q. So how is it done?**

**A.** I'm afraid it's a bit technical. Earlier in the book I explained that free radicals have a single unpaired electron in the outer orbital. The pair of electrons in other, closed, orbitals spin in opposite directions and thus the magnetic fields caused by the moving electron charges cancel each other. The unpaired electron, however, creates an unopposed magnetic field. Electron spin resonance is a method of detecting changes of spin in unpaired electrons in a powerful magnetic field that are exposed to microwave radio signals, much in the manner of the MRI scanner. A single electron in a strong magnetic field must be oriented either with or against the field. The two orientations differ slightly in energy and the radio signals can cause the occasional electron to flip from the lower to the higher energy state. On returning to its lower energy state the electron gives off a signal that can be detected.

**Q. There seems to be some evidence that fields from electric power lines and transformers can cause cancer. Could a free radical with its unpaired electron be affected by such fields?**

**A.** Yes. Very weak fields of the strength caused by power lines, etc., could move free radicals and, at least in theory, might interfere with pairs of radicals with opposite electron spin hooking up with each other to form a safe, non-active pair. If this happened on a large scale, there would be far more free radicals about than normal and this could lead to cancer. This is all completely theoretical and I don't think there has been any proof that this actually happens. Also, don't forget that all of us have been exposed to the earth's magnetic field from the time of conception. Maybe the interaction of the fixed field of the earth and the alternating field from power lines could have undesirable effects. The chemist, Keith McLauchlan, of Oxford University published a paper on this in January 1992 in *Physics World.*

**Q. Why do textbooks of nutrition recommend doses of vitamins C and E that are so much smaller than those you are recommending?**

**A.** The textbooks are concerned simply with avoiding the vitamin-deficiency diseases. Few have yet got around to recognizing the value of antioxidant vitamins as general health measures. This is a different use of these vitamins.

**Q. So would it be a good thing to take much larger doses of vitamin D and the B vitamins?**

**A.** On no account should you take large doses of vitamin D (or of vitamin A for that matter). Both would be dangerous (see p. 80). The B vitamins are not antioxidants. They are coenzymes, needed to allow various body enzyme systems to work, and are needed in very small quantities. You will get no advantage from taking larger doses than the recommended minimum daily allowances and you will get these from a decent balanced diet.

**Q. Is taking beta-carotene the same as taking vitamin A?**

**A.** Not quite. Although the two are closely related chemically, beta-carotene has been shown to have value against free radicals in certain conditions in which vitamin A seems ineffective. Beta-carotene is, however, the main human source of vitamin A and is soon converted by the liver into vitamin A, but this takes different forms with different functions. One form (retinal) is necessary for vision, others (retinol, retinoic acid, etc.) are necessary for healthy surface tissues (epithelia), and so on.

**Q. Isn't it possible that free radicals are just a by-product of other much more important disease processes going on in the body?**

**A.** It's possible. But even the little that is known today about free radicals answers a great many questions that could not be answered before. That knowledge is consistent with a lot of established facts. There is a principle in logic, highly regarded by medical and other scientists, called 'Occam's razor'. This states that a single explanation that accounts for a whole lot of apparently unrelated facts is more likely to be right than a lot of different explanations. Unifying principles of this kind have been immensely fruitful throughout the history of science. I rather suspect that the enormous importance of free radicals in medicine is going to be another one.

# Glossary

**Acne** A common skin disease of adolescence and early adult life, affecting white people and featuring blackheads, pimples and scarring.

**Addiction** Dependence on the repeated use of a drug such as nicotine, alcohol or heroin for comfort of mind or body.

**Aflatoxin** A poison produced by the fungus, *Aspergillus flavus*, which grows on peanuts and grains stored in damp conditions, and which can cause liver cancer.

**AIDS** The acquired immune deficiency syndrome, caused by the human immunodeficiency virus (HIV).

**Alpha-tocopherol** Vitamin E.

**Anaemia** A reduction in the amount of the oxygen-carrying substance, haemoglobin, in the blood.

**Aneurysm** A berry-like or diffuse swelling on an *artery*, usually at or near a branch, and caused by weakness in the artery wall, commonly from *atherosclerosis.*

**Angina pectoris** The symptom of oppression,

pain or tightness in the centre of the chest which occurs when the coronary *arteries* are unable to provide an adequate blood supply to meet the demands of the heart muscle.

**Angiography** — A form of X-ray examination using a fluid opaque to X-rays which renders the blood visible in blood vessels into which it has been injected.

**Antioxidant** — A substance capable of preventing the *oxidation* of organic *molecules*. A substance, such as vitamin C or vitamin E, capable of neutralizing or 'mopping up' damaging *free radicals*.

**Aorta** — The main *artery* of the body that arises directly from the heart and supplies branches to all parts.

**Aromatic hydrocarbon** — An organic compound containing a ring of six carbon *atoms* joined by alternating single and double *bonds*.

**Artery** — An elastic, muscular-walled tube carrying blood at high pressure from the heart to any part of the body.

**Atherosclerosis** — A degenerative disease of *arteries* in which fatty plaques develop on the inner lining of arteries so that the normal flow of blood is impeded. It is the major cause of death in the Western world and is responsible for more deaths than any other single condition.

**Atom** The smallest quantity of an *element* that can take part in a chemical reaction.

**Balloon angioplasty** The use of a *balloon catheter* to restore more normal width to an *artery* narrowed by *atherosclerosis.*

**Balloon catheter** A fine double tube, with an expandable cylindrical inflatable portion near one end, that can be passed along an *artery* to an area partially blocked by disease and inflated so as to crush the atherosclerotic plaque into the wall and widen the vessel.

**Benign** Not malignant. Mild, not usually tending to cause death.

**Beta-carotene** The orange pigment in carrots and other vegetables that is converted to vitamin A by the liver. It is a powerful *antioxidant.*

**BHA** See entry *butylated hydroxyanisole.*

**BHT** See entry *butylated hydroxytoluene.*

| | |
|---|---|
| **Bile duct** | The tube leading from the liver to the intestine down which bile passes. |
| **Bonds** | The chemical linkages between *atoms* joining to form *molecules.* |
| **Brain damage** | Any permanent loss of full brain function, however caused. |
| **Bronchiole** | One of the small air tubes of the lungs. |
| **Butyl-alpha-phenylni-trone** | An *antioxidant* substance that has been used experimentally to prevent *free radical* damage. |
| **Butylated hydroxyanisole** | An *antioxidant* widely used as an additive to preserve food. |
| **Butylated hydroxytoluene** | An *antioxidant* widely used as a food preservative. |
| **Calcification** | The laying down of chalky material in living tissues. |
| **Carcinogen** | Anything that can cause cancer. |
| **Carcinoma** | A cancer of surface *cells* – the commonest class of cancers. |
| **Carotenoids** | A group of pigments related to vitamin A. |
| **Carotid** | One of the two main *arteries* on the side of the neck that carry blood up to the brain. |
| **Catalase** | An *enzyme* that breaks down |

*hydrogen peroxide* into water and oxygen.

| | |
|---|---|
| **Cataract** | Any opacification of the internal lens of the eye. |
| **Cell** | The structural and functional unit of all living things. |
| **Cerebral haemorrhage** | Bleeding into the brain. |
| **Ceruloplasmin** | One of the body's natural *antioxidants.* |
| **Chemical reaction** | Any process in which *atoms* form linkages or linked atoms separate. |
| **Chemistry** | The science of the composition, properties and reactions of substances. |
| **Cholesterol** | An essential fatty sterol found in all body tissues, especially in *cell* membranes, that is also used by the body to synthesize other steroid substances. |
| **Compound** | A substance containing *atoms* of two or more *elements* held together by chemical *bonds.* |
| **Congenital malformation** | Any bodily abnormality present at birth. |
| **Conjunctiva** | The transparent membrane that covers the white of the eye and the inside of the eyelids. |

| | |
|---|---|
| **Contact inhibition** | The restraint on *cell* reproduction caused by contact with adjacent cells. |
| **Cornea** | The transparent front lens of the eye. |
| **Coronary arteries** | The two *arteries* that arise from the *aorta* and divide to form branches that spread over the surface of the heart to supply the constantly contracting muscle with blood. The left coronary artery divides into two near its origin, so it is reasonable to say that there are three coronary arteries. |
| **Coronary thrombosis** | Clotting of blood in a coronary *artery* of the heart, almost always at the site of an atherosclerotic plaque. |
| **Crystalline lens** | The internal lens of the eye that lies just behind the coloured iris. |
| **Cysteine** | A sulphur-containing amino acid (*protein* building-block). |
| **D-penicillamine** | One of the body's natural *antioxidants*. |
| **Dementia** | Progressive loss of mind, commonly the result of *atherosclerosis* of the *arteries* supplying the brain. |
| **Dermatologist** | A skin specialist. |

| | |
|---|---|
| **Detoxication** | A chemical change that renders a poisonous substance safer. |
| **DNA** | Deoxyribonucleic acid. The double-helix *molecule* that contains the genetic code blueprint for the structure of all the body *proteins*. |
| **Dopamine** | An important chemical found in the brain that can carry information and that is used to form adrenaline. |
| **Dupuytren's contracture** | A tightening of the fibrous layer below the skin of the palm of the hand so that the fingers are left permanently and fixedly bent. |
| **Electron** | The tiny negatively-charged particle on the outside of *atoms* that forms the linkages in chemical *bonds* and whose unbalanced presence forms a *free radical.* |
| **Electron paramagnetic resonance spectroscopy** | An advanced technique for detecting the presence of *free radicals.* |
| **Element** | One of the 92 naturally occurring substances of which the universe is made. Elements contain only one kind of *atom* and cannot be broken down further by chemical means. |
| **Empirical treatment** | Treatment without an explanatory basis. |

**Emulsifier** Any agent that allows oil and water to mix thoroughly to form a milky liquid.

**Endonuclease** An *enzyme* that can cut *DNA* at any specific point within the double helix.

**Enzyme** A *protein* capable of greatly accelerating the rate of an organic chemical reaction.

**Epidermis** The outer layer of the skin.

**Epithelium** A layer of *cells*, covering any internal or external surface of the body, that prevents body tissues from healing together.

**Exonucleases** *Enzymes* that can cut a length of *DNA* from a free end.

**Fetus** The human embryo from about the second month of pregnancy to the time of birth. Note that the spelling 'foetus' is incorrect.

**Fibroblasts** *Cells* that form the collagen *protein* – the main constituent of fibrous tissue.

**Flavonoids** A group of organic compounds that form the colouring matter of plants and flowers.

**Free radical** An *atom* or group of atoms with an unpaired *electron*, forming a chemically highly active agent avid to latch on to any nearby *molecule* and to oxidize it. Free radicals are so active that most of them persist only for very short periods before being inactivated on attacking another molecule. In so doing, however, they can convert the second molecule into a free radical and thus start a damaging chain reaction. Free radicals can be tamed and preserved for research purposes by freezing with liquid nitrogen.

**French paradox** — The surprisingly low incidence of *atherosclerosis* in a population with a high dietary intake of saturated fats.

**Gangrene** — Death of tissue.

**Gerontology** — The science of ageing.

**Glucose** — A simple sugar, the main fuel of the body.

**Glucose-6-phosphate dehydrogenase** — An *enzyme* important in carbohydrate usage in the body. Deficiency causes a form of *anaemia*.

**Glutathione** — One of the body's natural *antioxidants*.

**Heart attack** — Death of a segment of the heart muscle as a result of *coronary thrombosis* or coronary spasm that cuts off the blood supply to the muscle.

**Heart failure** — The point at which the heart is no longer able to keep the blood circulating adequately, so that stagnation occurs with fluid accumulation in the tissues.

**High-density lipoproteins** — Complexes of fats and *proteins*, with a preponderance of the latter, that move *cholesterol* from the body tissues to the liver. These are the beneficial lipoproteins.

**HIV positive** — Having antibodies to the human immunodeficiency virus.

**Hormones** — Chemical messengers that help to control and coordinate various body and cellular functions.

**Hydrogen peroxide** — A *molecule* similar to that of water but containing an additional oxygen *atom* so that it is a strong oxidizing agent.

**Hydroxyl ion** — One of the two parts into which the water *molecule* naturally splits.

**Hydroxyl radical** — A highly active *free radical* consisting of a hydrogen *atom* and an oxygen atom with a single unpaired *electron.*

**Hypoxanthine** — A substance formed when nucleoproteins (*proteins* bound to nucleic acid as in *DNA*) are broken down, as by *free radicals.*

**Inflammation** The body's response to injury. Local blood supply increases and *cells* of the immune system, such as *phagocytes*, are brought to the site.

**Intravenous** Within a vein.

**Ion** An electrically charged *atom* or group of atoms formed when an *electron* is gained or lost.

**Iris** The coloured part of the eye with a central hole, the pupil.

**Junk DNA** *DNA* that does not carry genetic information.

**LDLs** See entry *low-density lipoproteins.*

**Lentigines** Large age-related freckles on the skin. The singular is 'lentigo'.

**Leukaemia** A kind of cancer of the blood-forming tissues in the bone marrow in which a great excess of abnormal white blood *cells* is produced so that the blood cannot properly perform its vital functions.

**Lipids** Fats.

**Liver** The main site of biochemical activity in the body.

| | |
|---|---|
| **Low-density lipoproteins** | Complexes of fats and *proteins*, with a preponderance of the former, that move from the liver to the body tissues. These are the damaging lipoproteins. |
| **Malignancy** | Having a tendency to cause death or serious bodily disorder. |
| **Malignant melanoma** | A cancer of the skin-colouring *cells* – the melanocytes. |
| **Malonaldehyde** | A substance released in the course of high levels of tissue *oxidation* and thus serving as a marker of *free radical* activity. |
| **Metabolic rate** | The speed with which the bodily chemical processes occur. |
| **Metabolism** | The totality of the chemical processes occurring in the body and resulting in growth, tissue breakdown, the production of energy, the disposal of unwanted substances, and so on. Metabolism includes build-up (anabolism) and breakdown (catabolism). |
| **Metastasis** | Remote spread of cancer by seeding out of small groups of cancer *cells* conveyed by the blood or the lymph. |
| **Micrometastases** | Inapparent transmission of microscopic groups of cancer *cells*. |

**Micronuclei** Fragments of *DNA* released into the *cell* fluids after *free radical* and other damage.

**Mitochondria** Small spherical or rod-like bodies in *cells* that contain *enzymes* responsible for energy production and a circular genome of *DNA*.

**Molecule** The smallest unit of a chemical compound, consisting of two or more *atoms* bound together by chemical *bonds*. Some molecules, such as those of *protein*, are very large.

**Mutation** A change in *DNA* that damages or alters its genetic effect.

**Naphthols** A group of *antioxidant* substances.

**Night blindness** Poor vision in dim light, as occurs in vitamin A deficiency.

**Nitrosamines** A class of oily compounds containing the group NNO. They can occur during the overcooking of meats and are thought to be able to cause cancer.

**Oesophagus** The gullet, down which food passes to the stomach.

**Oncogenes** Genes that can activate *DNA* in

such a way as to turn the *cell* cancerous.

**Osteomalacia** — Softening of the bones in adults from calcium deficiency secondary to vitamin D deficiency.

**Oxidation** — The process of undergoing a combination with oxygen or of suffering a loss of *electrons*. Oxidation is often destructive, as in rusting or burning, but is an essential part of the process of releasing energy in the body and elsewhere.

**Oxidative stress** — A term widely used to refer to the action of *free radicals*.

**Paediatrician** — A specialist in child medicine.

**PBN** — See entry *butyl-alpha-phenylnitrone*.

**Peroxidation** — A chemical reaction, stimulated in the body by poisons and infections, in which oxygen *atoms* are freed and then attached to *molecules* such as that of water to form substances capable of strong *oxidation*.

**Phagocytes** — Scavenging *cells* of the immune system that engulf and destroy germs and unwanted material by forming *free radicals*.

**Phenol** — Carbolic acid, one of a class of

compounds containing a benzene ring and a hydroxyl group.

**Phenolic** — Containing, or derived from, phenol.

**Photo-ageing** — The damaging effect on skin of long-term exposure to light.

**Plaques** — The term used for the raised mounds of degenerate muscle *cells* and *cholesterol* that form on the inner lining of *arteries* in the diseasc of *atherosclerosis.*

**Polyunsaturated fats** — Fats containing fatty acids in which many of the carbon linkages have double *bonds* and are thus more easily broken than the more stable single bonds. Unsaturated fats are usually liquid at room temperature.

**Prospective studies** — Trials, as of the value of *antioxidant* supplements, in which the conditions are set before the trials begin and the results are assessed in the future.

**Protein** — The main constructional and functional material of the body, formed by the linkage of various combinations of 20 amino acids into large *molecules*. Proteins may be soluble, as in the case of the blood proteins, antibodies and *enzymes*, or insoluble as in the case of the collagen of bones and connective tissue and the keratin of the hair and nails.

**Radical** A chemical group or associated cluster of *atoms* usually forming a part of a *molecule* that often retains its identity in the course of chemical reactions.

**Reperfusion** The renewed flow of blood into an area of the body after it has been cut off. This results from the opening up of nearby closed blood vessels and is commonly associated with intense action by *free radicals.*

**Replication** The process of exact copying, as occurs in *DNA* before *cell* reproduction.

**Retinol** Vitamin A.

**Retrolental fibroplasia** A serious and often blinding eye disorder occurring in premature babies given too much oxygen.

**Rickets** Bone softening and distortion occurring in infants deficient in vitamin D.

**Saturated fat** Fat containing fatty acids whose carbon *atom* linkages are all by single, and thus stable, *bonds.* Most saturated fats are solid at room temperature.

**Scurvy** The bleeding disorder from

defective synthesis of collagen caused by a severe deficiency of vitamin C.

| | |
|---|---|
| **Seminal fluid** | The sticky fluid containing millions of sperms that is emitted during sexual ejaculation. |
| **Stroke** | A serious disorder resulting from brain damage caused by deprivation of blood or bleeding into or around the brain. |
| **Substantia nigra** | A darkly pigmented part of the brain that produces the substance, *dopamine*. |
| **Superoxide** | A metal oxide containing an oxygen *ion*. One of the most important *free radicals* formed in the body, that can attack fats, *proteins* and carbohydrates. |
| **Superoxide dismutase** | One of the body's natural *antioxidants*, capable of inactivating the *superoxide free radical.* |
| **Telangiectasis** | 'Broken veins'. |
| **Telomeres** | The end segments of the *DNA* of chromosomes. |
| **Thrombosis** | Clotting of blood within an *artery* or a vein. |
| **Tissue** | Any collection of joined *cells.* |

| | |
|---|---|
| **Tissue culture** | The artificial growth of sheets of body *cells*, such as fibroblasts, in glass dishes in the laboratory. |
| **Tocopherol** | Vitamin E. |
| **Tocopherols** | A group of compounds related to or constituting vitamin E. |
| **Transferrin** | One of the body's natural *antioxidants.* |
| **Transient ischaemic attack / TIA** | A mini-stroke lasting for less than 24 hours. TIAs are serious warnings that a full stroke, with permanent damage, may occur at any time. |
| **Tretinoin** | The active form of vitamin A in all body tissues except the retina of the eye. |
| **Ulceration** | A breakdown of any body surface to form a crater and expose the underlying *tissue*. |
| **Ultraviolet light / radiation** | The part of the electromagnetic spectrum that lies between visible light and X-rays. Most of the sun's UVL is filtered out by the atmosphere, but it is still capable of provoking much *free radical* formation in the skin. |
| **Xanthine** | A substance involved in the production of *free radicals*, that can act as a marker of free radical activity. |

# Further Reading


'Alzheimer's disease and free radicals', *British Medical Journal*, 23 March 1996, p. 728.

'Antioxidant herbal remedies', *Journal of the Royal Society of Medicine*, September 1996, p. 540.

'Antioxidant in tea cuts heart attacks 75%', *Lancet*, 8 March 1997, p. 735.

'Antioxidant vitamins and colorectal cancer', *New England Journal of Medicine*, 22 December 1994, p. 1720.

'Antioxidant state and heart attacks', *British Medical Journal*, 1 March 1997, pp. 629, 634.

'Antioxidants and atherosclerosis', *Lancet*, 1 July 1995, p. 36.

'Antioxidants, chocolate, phenolics, flavonoids', *Lancet*, 21 September 1996, p. 834.

'Antioxidants and dementia, vitamins C and E', *Lancet*, 26 April 1997, p. 1188.

'Antioxidants and heart disease', *New England Journal of Medicine*, 2 May 1996, pp. 1145, 1150, 1156, 1189.

'Antioxidants for ischaemic heart disease', *Lancet*, 14 June 1997, pp. 1710, 1715.

'Antioxidants, free radicals, vitamin C', *New Scientist*, 7 October 1989, p. 29.

'Antioxidants and disease mechanisms', *New England Journal of Medicine*, 7 August 1997, p. 408.

'Antioxidants and phytotherapy', *Lancet*, 12 November 1994, p. 1356.

'Atherosclerosis, oxidation, free radicals', *Lancet*, 12 November 1994, p. 1363.

'Atherosclerosis and oxidation, free radicals', *Lancet*, 17 September 1994, p. 793.

'Beta-carotene, càncer and heart disease trials', *Lancet*, 27 January 1996, p. 249.

'Beta-carotene as preventive for cancer', *New England Journal of Medicine*, 3 October 1996, p. 1065.

Chronic obstructive lung disease and antioxidants', *British Medical Journal*, 14 January 1995, p. 75.

'Claudication and Padma-28 antioxidants', *Lancet*, 2 April 1994, p. 847.

'Cooked tomatoes attack free radicals', *Lancet*, 25 October 1997, p. 1229.
'Drug gingko biloba, dementia, free radicals', *Lancet*, 25 October 1997, p. 1229.
'Dupuytren's in HIV patients, free radicals', *British Medical Journal*, 20 January 1990.
'Effect of fruit and vegetable intake on lipids', *British Medical Journal*, 21 June 1997, p. 1787.
'Factors in ageing, free radicals, radiation', *Journal of the Royal Society of Medicine*, 3 September 1994, p. 540.
'Flavonoids and heart disease, free radicals', *British Medical Journal*, 24 February 1996, pp. 458, 478.
'Free radicals and G-6 phosphate dehydrogenase', *British Medical Journal*, 27 March 1993, p. 841.
'Free radicals editorial', *New England Journal of Medicine*, 14 April 1994, p. 1080.
'Free radicals, antioxidants, lung, prostate cancer', *New England Journal of Medicine*, 14 April 1994, p. 1029.
'Free radicals, heart disease, vitamin E', *New England Journal of Medicine*, 20 May 1993, pp. 1444–56,1487.
'Free radicals, antioxidants, heart attack', *Lancet*, 4 December 1993, p. 1379.
'Free radicals, diet after coronary thrombosis', *British Medical Journal*, 18 April 1993, p. 1015.
'Free radicals, flavonoids, coronary disease', *Lancet*, 23 October 1993, p. 1007.
'Free radicals and neurodegenerative disease', *Lancet*, 17 September 1994, p. 796.
'Free radicals and malnutrition', *New Scientist*, 17 February 1990, p. 38.
'Free radicals in health and disease', *British Journal of Hospital Medicine*, May 1990, p. 334.
'Free radicals, smoking and sperm', *New Scientist*, 6 March 1993, p. 10.
'Free radicals, tocopherol and Parkinson's disease, *New England Journal of Medicine*, 21 January 1993, p. 176.
'Free radicals and vascular disease', *British Medical Journal*, 9 October 1993, p. 885.
'Free radicals, vitamin A and cancer in China', *New Scientist*, 22 May 1993, p. 7.

'Free radicals in medicine, book review', *British Medical Journal*, 10 September 1994, p. 678.

'Free radicals, red wine, antioxidant LDL', *Lancet*, 20 February 1993, p. 454.

'Free radicals, antioxidants, full review', *Lancet*, 10 September 1994, pp. 721, 722.

'Free radicals, vitamins, breast cancer', *New England Journal of Medicine*, 18 November 1993, p. 1579.

'Free radicals, antioxidants and coronary disease', *Journal of the American Medical Association*, 19 December 1990, p. 3049.

'Free radicals and wine', *Lancet*, 2 January 1993, p. 27.

'Free radicals and cataract', *British Medical Journal*, 5 December 1992, p. 1392.

'Free radicals and cancer', *Lancet*, 24 September 1994, p. 862.

'Free radicals and pressure sores', *British Medical Journal*, 5 December 1992, p. 1433.

'Free radicals and the lung', *Lancet*, 1 October 1994, p. 930.

'Free radicals and antioxidants in bowel disease', *Lancet*, 24 September 1994, p. 859.

'Free radicals and antioxidants', *Lancet*, 19 November 1994, p. 1440.

'Free radicals and angina', *Lancet*, 5 January 1991, p. 1.

'Free radicals and RDS', *Lancet*, 27 March 1993, p. 777.

'Free radicals and smoking', *Science*, 18 December 1992, p. 1875.

'Free radicals ageing protein oxidation', *Science*, 28 August 1992, p. 1220.

'Free radicals, vitamins E and A and stroke', *Lancet*, 27 June 1992, p. 1562.

'Free radicals', *New Scientist*, 11 August 1988, p. 41.

'Free radicals', *Journal of the Royal Society of Medicine*, December 1989, p. 747.

'Free radicals vascular disease', *British Medical Journal*, 17 June 1995, pp. 1548, 1559, 1563.

'Free radicals', *British Journal of Hospital Medicine*, 4 November 1992, p. 591.

'Free radicals, diabetes and low vitamin E levels', *British Medical Journal*, 28 October 1995, p. 1124.

'Free radicals, vitamin A and child mortality', *Journal of the American Medical Association*, 17 February 1993, p. 898.

'Free radicals, vitamin E heart disease', *New England Journal of Medicine*, 4 November 1993, p. 1426.
'Free radicals and heart attack', *Lancet*, 17 April 1993, p. 990.
'Free radicals, vitamin C and cognitive function in age', *British Medical Journal*, 9 March 1996, p. 608.
'Free radicals, pre-eclampsia oxidized LDLs', *Lancet*, 12 March 1994, p. 645.
'Free radicals and oral cancer prevention', *Lancet*, 6 November 1993, p. 1129.
'Free radicals, vitamins and breast cancer', *New England Journal of Medicine*, 22 July 1993, p. 234.
'Free radicals can also fight cancers', *New Scientist*, 13 September 1997, p. 16.
'French paradox wine, diet, heart disease', *Lancet*, 24 December 1994, p. 1719.
'HRT and atherosclerosis antioxidant', *Lancet*, 14 January 1995, p. 76.
'Lung cancer and antioxidant vitamins', *New England Journal of Medicine*, 1 September. 1994, p. 611.
'Molecular sex and free radicals', *New Scientist*, 22 October 1994, p. 45.
'Oxidative damage in diabetes free radicals', *Lancet*, 17 February 1996, p. 444.
'Padma-28 antioxidants', *Lancet*, 12 November 1994, p. 1356.
'Phagocytes and free radicals', *British Journal of Clinical Practice*, February 1990, p. 45.
'Reperfusion injury after heart attack, free radicals', *British Medical Journal*, 25 February 1995, p. 477.
'Smoking and free radicals antioxidants', *New England Journal of Medicine*, 4 May 1995, p. 1198.
'Tea flavonoids and antioxidant activity', *British Medical Journal*, 27 July 1996, p. 229.
'Vitamin E enhances immune system, antioxidants', *British Medical Journal*, 10 May 1997, p. 1369.
'Vitamin C and the brain, antioxidants', *Journal of the Royal Society of Medicine*, May 1996, p. 241.
'Vitamin E, antioxidant free radicals', *Lancet*, 21 January 1995, p. 170.
'Vitamin E, heart protection in diabetes', *British Medical Journal*, 28 June 1997, p. 1845.
'Volatile organic compounds, free radicals', *New Scientist*, 21 June 1997, p. 30.

# Index

□□□